Topographic Labiaplasty

Pablo Gonzalez-Isaza • Rafael Sánchez-Borrego

Editors

Topographic Labiaplasty

From Theory to Clinical Practice

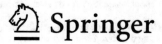

Editors
Pablo Gonzalez-Isaza (iD)
Obstetrics and Gynecology Urogynecology
Minimally Invasive Surgery Functional
Cosmetic and Regenerative Gynecology
Hospital Universitario San Jorge/Liga
contra el Cancer
Pereira, Madrid, Spain

Rafael Sánchez-Borrego (iD)
Gynaecology and Obstetrics Department
DIATROS Woman'sClinic
Barcelona, Barcelona, Spain

The translation was done with the help of artificial intelligence (machine translation by the service DeepL.com). A subsequent human revision was done primarily in terms of content.

ISBN 978-3-031-15050-0   ISBN 978-3-031-15048-7   (eBook)
https://doi.org/10.1007/978-3-031-15048-7

This Springer imprint is published by the registered company Springer Nature Switzerland AG
The registered company address is: Gewerbestrasse 11, 6330 Cham, Switzerland

To my wife Heidi Fruchtnis, my daughter Julieta Gonzalez, a permanent source of inspiration, they have been a witness to my professional career, to my parents who have allowed me to have a quality education, to my colleagues and friends who experience the great satisfaction of improving the sexuality and quality of life of patients.

Pablo Gonzalez-Isaza

Foreword

Many years ago, I had the opportunity to contact Dr. Pablo Gonzalez through a colleague who introduced us. We met at a conference in Bogota, and there for the first time I learned about some of the procedures of cosmetic gynecology. At that time, there was a lot of resistance from some positions—not so much theoretical or scientific but ideological—from sexual health professionals, and I found it interesting to dive deeper into the subject to have my own concept of the subject.

Shortly thereafter, I participated in the first Cosmetic Gynecology congress in the city of Pereira, and there I heard brilliant presentations from different doctors that made me understand that this is a science, and not a deceptive practice. Behind those conferences, there was the support of well-designed research, scientific publications, books, hundreds of operating room hours, and international scientific societies.

At this point is where we understand the difference between science and ideology, two perspectives that do not always speak the same language. And I think that not only from science but also from common sense a woman has every right in the world to have some kind of aesthetic intervention that allows her to feel more comfortable with her body, increase her self-esteem, overcome complexes, and fully enjoy her sexuality. In summary, it is her body, and not even radical feminist groups have more right than her to make the corresponding decisions.

In the following years, we continued to strength our professional relationship in different congresses, meetings, courses, and I observed the exponential growth of cosmetic gynecology, something that perhaps I would not have known about if it had not been for that first providential meeting.

My now friend Pablo Gonzalez was always concerned about being at the forefront, organizing large conferences, teaching, writing, publishing, and of course performing surgical procedures. But he still had something pending: to publish a book.

So, the time came, with some texts of his authorship and chapters of world-renowned professionals, he built this dream named: *Topographic Labiaplasty: From theory to practice*. Its contents, as its title suggests, range from historical, theoretical and, of course, practical aspects that give a complete picture of labiaplasty from a scientific perspective.

I have no doubt that this book will make history within the specialty, and I hope it will have the reception and repercussion it deserves. It has plenty of quality to achieve it. Enjoy it.

Private Practice   Ezequiel López Peralta
Bogota, Colombia

Contents

Chapter 1
Introduction

Pablo Gonzalez-Isaza

Introduction

Labia minora hypertrophy, usually, is of multifactorial origin; it can be considered as an anatomical variant [1–4] or due to genetic alterations as reported in the current literature in studies with identical twins [5], by the accidental administration of androgens in pregnancy, by mechanical factors such as chronic irritation, neurodegenerative diseases such as myelodysplasia, adrenal hyperplasia, childbirth, lymphatic stasis, irritations, and chronic inflammation due to urinary incontinence. It has been described in some sexual habits such as the use of piercing, by the intentional stretching of the labia minora known in the African cultures of Khoikhoi, Hottentot tribe, among other [5, 6], and finally mentioned in some series without further support by excessive masturbation, or it simply can be classified as idiopathic origin, in general terms, which should be considered as a variant of normal anatomy.

Hypertrophy is defined as the disproportionate size of the labia minora with respect to the labia majora; it should be noted that the elongation of tissues in the vulva may have multiple components affecting not only the labia minora but also the clitoral hood, vestibule, and perianal region [7].

Among the most frequent reasons for consultation, we can find difficulty in managing vaginal secretions, vulvovaginitis, and chronic irritation as well as mass sensation and functional limitation for performing sports activities, such as cycling or horseback riding [1, 4, 8, 9], superficial dyspareunia, and secondary sexual dysfunction are frequent; it has also been reported the entrapment of the labia minora in the closure of the garments. They are generally patients who have a very important

P. Gonzalez-Isaza (✉)
Obstetrics and Gynecology Urogynecology Minimally Invasive Surgery Functional Cosmetic and Regenerative Gynecology, Hospital Universitario San Jorge/Liga contra el Cancer, Pereira, Madrid, Spain

© The Author(s), under exclusive license to Springer Nature Switzerland AG 2023
P. Gonzalez-Isaza, R. Sánchez-Borrego (eds.), *Topographic Labiaplasty*, https://doi.org/10.1007/978-3-031-15048-7_1

psychosocial component due to the alteration in their self-esteem and the impossibility of leading a satisfactory intimate life [6].

In most cases, despite of an adequate counseling to these patients, the management is surgical, with labiaplasty or nymphoplasty [10–13].

The main objective of this procedure is the resection of hypertrophic tissue, achieving a functional and cosmetic impact for these patients [8, 9, 14]. Multiple techniques have been described, ranging from a simple resection under local anesthesia to the use of devices with different types of energy, mainly multipulsed CO_2 laser, which has shown the best results to date [15, 16].

Radmann et al. in their series of adolescent patients, considered hypertrophy to labia minora with a length greater than 5 cm the degrees of hypertrophy, but in general it is said that the labia minora that protrude outside the labia majora and have a length greater than 5 ms can be categorized as hypertrophic [7].

The proposal of topographic labiaplasty is a compilation of experiences of more than 14 years performing labiaplasty, which allowed to understand the great anatomical variability and complexity of the anatomy of the vulva, finally achieving a simple, reproducible, and safe technique for the approach of patients with labia minora hypertrophy; by reading this book, the reader will be able to easily understand and comprehend the approach to this type of patients.

References

1. Radman HM. Hypertrophy of the labia minora. Obstet Gynecol. 1976;48(1 Suppl):78S–9S.
2. Friedrich EG. Vulvar disease. 2nd ed. Philadelphia: Saunders; 1983.
3. Rouzzier R, Louis S, Paniel C. Hypertrophy of labia minora: experience with 163 reductions. Am J Obstet Gynecol. 2000;182(1 PT 1):35–40.
4. Pardo J, Sola V, Ricci P, Guilloff E. Laser labioplasty of the labia minora. Int J Gynaecol Obstet. 2006;93:38–43.
5. Galvin WJ. Labia Minora hypertrophy: a new surgical approach. Adolesc Pediatr Gynecol. 1995;8:39–42.
6. Paarlberg KM, Weijenborg PTM. Request for operative reduction of the labia minora; a proposal for practical guidelines for gynecologists. J Psychosom Obstet Gynecol. 2008;29:230–4.
7. Peter C, Mark S, Thomas N. Vaginal labiaplasty: defense of the simple "Clip and snip" and a new classification system. Aesthetic Plast Surg. 2013;37:887–9.
8. Maas SM, Hage JJ. Functional and aesthetic labia minora reduction. Plastic Reconstr Surg. 2000;105(14):53–6.
9. Jhansi R, Laufer R. Hypertrophy labia minora: mini review. J Pediatr Adolesc Gynecol. 2010;23:3–6.
10. Godmann M. Is elective vulvar plastic surgery ever warranted? And what screening should be conducted preoperatively? J Sex Med. 2007;4:269–76.
11. Koning M, Zeijlmans IA, Bouman T, van der Lei B. Female attitudes regarding labia minora appearance and reduction with consideration of media influence. Aesthet Surg J. 2009;29:65–71.
12. Chavis WM, LaFerla JJ, Niccolini R. Plastic repair of elongated, hypertrophic labia minora: a case report. J Reprod Med. 1989;34:373–5.
13. Lee PA, Witchel SF. Genital surgery among females with congenital adrenal hyperplasia: changes over the past five decades. J Pediatr Endocrinol Metab. 2002;15:1473–7.

14. Lynch A, Marulaiah M, Samarakkody U. Reduction labioplasty in adolescents. J Pediatr Adolesc Gynecol. 2008;3:147–9.
15. Ellsworth WA, Rivzi M, Lypka M. Techniques for labia minora reduction: an algorithmic approach. Aesthetic Plast Surg. 2010;34:105–10.
16. Liao L-M, Michala L, Creighton S. Labial surgery for well women: a review of the literature. BJOG. 2010;117:20–5.

Chapter 2
Historical Aspects

Jack Pardo Schanz

History of Labiaplasty

The labia minora and clitoral hood have a common embryological origin with the foreskin of the penis. The first surgery recorded in antiquity related to the genital area is inside the Bible, in Genesis, when God ordered the Prophet Abraham to circumcise his son Isaac and previously circumcised himself to formalize as God said: "A covenant between me and you [1]." In antiquity, for unknown reasons, but apparently related to decrease or abolish female sexual pleasure, female circumcision, or female genital mutilation (FGM) began to be practiced initially in Ancient Egypt, which, depending on each culture, ranged from the removal of the clitoris alone to the so-called pharaonic circumcision [2], which consists of an almost total vulvectomy, removing the clitoris, its hood, and labia minora, besides closing almost completely the introitus. The practice of FGM is still carried out—unfortunately—even in the twenty-first century. Although it is mostly performed in Muslim countries, its origin predates the appearance of Muhammad by hundreds of years (sixth century), and current Muslim theologians consider it an unnecessary practice and contrary to Islam. I have referred to FGM in this chapter expressly to make it absolutely clear that it has no medical, cultural, or surgical relationship to any of the surgeries that comprise female genital aesthetics or cosmetogynecology. Moreover, leading cosmetogynecologists, such as Dr. Amr Seifeldin of Egypt, are experts in performing FGM repair surgery [3]. There are feminist movements, especially, and some medical societies that have tried to relate and even catalog female genital cosmetic and plastic surgery, mainly labiaplasty with FGM [4], nothing further from reality since the latter are aimed at improving the quality of life, sexuality, and genital aesthetics, which contrasts with FGM that is oriented to the opposite.

J. Pardo Schanz (✉)
Clinica Ginestetica, Santiago, Chile

P. Gonzalez-Isaza, R. Sánchez-Borrego (eds.), *Topographic Labiaplasty*,
https://doi.org/10.1007/978-3-031-15048-7_2

As for surgeries of the female external genitalia, we have very old citations of procedures performed by physicians.

Soranus of Ephesus (98–138 A.D.), a Greek physician who practiced in Alexandria and Rome in the late first and early second centuries, provides us with the first record of cosmetic genital surgery in history for an aesthetic defect [5]. He describes the excision of a hypertrophic clitoris for cosmetic reasons and to "decrease excessive sexual stimulation." In any case, he refers in this surgery to the procedure described by Philomenus, a contemporary of him. Later, another doctor, with the same name as the previous one, Philomenus of Alexandria, in the third century, also performed a partial clitoridectomy for hypertrophic clitoris because he considered it "ugly" [6].

Continuing the timeline in the seventh century, Paulus of Aegina, physician of the Byzantine Empire, described two different operations, one of which was a partial clitoridectomy and the second a partial resection of the labia minora which he called "cauda pudenda" (pudendal tail) [7].

Although this operation may have been performed many times in the following centuries, it is not until the sixteenth century that François Mauriceau, a great French obstetrician–gynecologist of the time, in his treaty on "The Diseases of Women" [8], describes the nymphae or labia minora as "small membranous wings" whose purpose is to protect the vaginal entrance and, surprisingly, explains how they help to conduct the urinary stream correctly so that it does not disperse down the thighs. This is remarkable since all of us who perform labia minora labiaplasty know that total amputation of the labia minora in women with very flat labia majora produces this undesirable effect on urination. Mauriceau tells how some women have such large labia minora that for convenience they are forced to place them inside the labia majora. He relates the case of a young lady who was in severe discomfort because of her large labia minora and also because they affected her especially in equestrian activity. He operated on his patient performing a reductive labiaplasty and achieving the necessary success for the lady to be able to ride again. Another interesting fact is that he explains that "the labia minora are red and evolve to a darker color with age."

Later, Pierre Dionis, a Parisian surgeon described the excision of the nymphae (labia minora) in his treatise *Cours d'operation de chirugie* in 1707 based on his experience assisting the nobility of the court of Louis XIV, the Sun King. The military surgeon, Lorenz Heister, first described the labia minora in detail in his 1739 publication, *Institutiones Chirurgicae*, which is considered one of the most popular surgical atlases of the seventeenth century. He explains in detail: "The nymphs of women are sometimes very long, not only hang outside the labia (majora) but cause discomfort in walking, sitting, and sexual intercourse, and may require the assistance of a surgeon. The operator must sit in front of the patient in a suitable position, take the lip with his left hand and cut what he considers necessary using scissors with his right hand, having at hand preparations that help control bleeding and medications that prevent the patient from fainting. When the surgery is over, the wound should be treated with some kind of ointments and will heal without much difficulty with common methods. It is noteworthy that it does not mention any type of suture, which is not so incredible, since it is described that a labiaplasty can be performed without sutures."

During the following centuries, labiaplasty is reported sporadically. Apparently, it was not given the importance it deserved, but we can be sure that in important cases of labia minora hypertrophy, if the patient dared to consult and if the surgeon was kind, it can be assumed that this surgery was performed constantly over time, but without giving it the importance it deserved to be published in the medical literature in a scientific manner, so, during my residency at the Hospital del Salvador in Santiago de Chile between 1988 and 1993, I saw only one labiaplasty. In my last year of residency, without ever having seen a case, my direct boss, a renowned gynecological surgeon, asked me to perform a "nymphoplasty" after a hysterectomy that we had scheduled, as when after a major gynecological surgery biopsy scraping wase left for the gynecology resident. I only remember performing it with scissors and suturing step by step to immediately stop the bleeding. I have no memory of having a complication or the final result. That was to this day the only labiaplasty I have ever performed in my life, with traditional surgical instruments, and as of writing this article in September 2020, I have performed over a thousand of these procedures.

Honoré et al., in 1978, described two cases of labiaplasty for bilateral hypertrophy. In 1983, Darryl Hodgkinson, published what is considered the first communication of labiaplasty. In it, he begins by describing the sociological and personal reasons that may lead a woman to request this procedure. He emphasizes gyms, sports, and even the greater influence of plastic surgeons in wanting to treat these cases. There he explains that labia surgeries in modern gynecology were reserved in practice almost exclusively to massive vulvar hypertrophies secondary to congenital adrenal hyperplasia. He notes that women of that time requested reduction of the labia minora for aesthetic as well as functional reasons. He describes, quite correctly in my opinion, how some patients also (or sometimes exclusively) request reduction of the clitoral hood, which he calls a "partial circumcision." As in this chapter, Hodgkinson refers to FGM from the historical point of view and highlights how in the "present day" of 1983 there were social and political movements aimed at the abolition of FGM, a situation which almost 40 years later has proved to be failed. Her communication is based on the description of three clinical cases, under general anesthesia in one case and one of the cases concomitant with breast surgery.

In the prestigious and traditional *American Journal of Obstetrics and Gynecology* in 2000, Rouzier et al., from France, published a series of 163 cases of labiaplasty, reporting excellent results and cataloguing the procedure as simple and with a high degree of patient satisfaction [9].

This was one of the first communications with an important series of cases.

During the 1980s and 1990s, the pornographic industry had a real exposure, especially when the internet became massified and the vulva began to be visualized in a much more in an explicit way, unlike the traditional exposure of the torso and buttocks of the 1960s and 1970s, led by *Playboy* magazine [10]. The breasts were already too exposed; they were not a novelty; it was the birth of the cult of the vulva. We cannot omit, in any way, the influence that pornography had in the massification of labiaplasty, and with this we can add the total hair removal of the female genitalia named "Brazilian waxing." This epilation method "style" which consists of removing all the hair from the pubis, labia majora, and perianal area, was born in the early 1990s in New York in a female beauty center whose owners were six Brazilian sisters known as the "J Sisters." They imposed the fashion of total hair removal that left only a small part of the pubis with some hair, only as a decorative effect, or sometimes not at all. As the vulvas were left bare of hair in their entirety, in the 1990s the road to the interest of beautifying women's external genitalia was being paved. Mile zero of this road is in Los Angeles, California, specifically in Beverly Hills.

In 1997, an American gynecologist from California, Dr. David Matlock began the routine practice of what he called and settled on as "vaginal rejuvenation" which was a modification of the traditional colpoperineoplasty for prolapse surgery. Matlock, as described in "his path" in Michael Goodman's book, devised a concept and method that he could pass on to other physicians, supported by the knowledge he gained from his patients and from having completed an MBA. Gradually he realized that a large percentage of women he performed vaginal rejuvenation on were also requesting labiaplasty. His procedure was perfected with the use of a diode laser, free edge excision technique, and clitoral hood removal when necessary. He called this labiaplasty, *Designer Laser Vaginoplasty*, DLV®, meaning "laser-assisted vagina design." Like Laser Vaginal Rejuvenation, LVR®, both were trademarked. In the United States, you cannot offer to do a DLV® or LVR® if you have not taken the course taught by David Matlock. From 2000 to 2020, more than 400 gynecologists, urologists, and plastic surgeons from all over the world have taken Matlock's course. This is where my story with this surgery begins.

In 2003, along with Dr. Vicente Solá, we created the Pelvic Floor and Gynecologic Plastic Surgery Unit of Clínica Las Condes; I went to Beverly Hills, California to attend the vaginal rejuvenation course given by David Matlock. At the beginning of the course, David told me: "In addition to vaginal rejuvenation, I am going to teach you something else that will give you great satisfaction," and so it was that, with animal models (a fresh pig's ear); we learned to use a diode laser and practice to do laser labiaplasty.

When I returned to Chile, both labiaplasty and vaginal rejuvenation became part of my regular practice and absolutely integrated with other surgeries. It was very common to correct urinary incontinence with a mid-urethral tape and to perform laser-assisted vaginal rejuvenation and/or laser-assisted labiaplasty on the same patient. In 2005 we published the first series of laser labiaplasty in the world literature with excellent results, where we also proposed a classification and described the reasons that women had for requesting the surgery [11]. This was in addition to the first communication of vaginal rejuvenation in the world literature that we presented in 2006. Until that time, cosmetogynecology was a discipline formally and habitually practiced almost exclusively by Matlock's disciples.

From 2006 onwards, contributions of lectures in some congresses of laser medicine began to take place, and later a small eruption of gynecology courses with special chapters of cosmetogynecology began to take place, among which I must mention the advanced vision of the Paraguayan and Uruguayan Societies of

Gynecology, who early on invited me to show my experience and perform teaching surgeries with the aim of adding this discipline to the practice of gynecology and, above all, urogynecology.

It always seemed important to me to combine cosmetogynecology with urogynecology, since the association of patients with urinary incontinence seeking vaginal rejuvenation and/or labiaplasty was extremely important, as we have described in different publications. In fact, we have even described a case of labiaplasty and vaginal rejuvenation concomitant with a radical hysterectomy for stage I cervical cancer.

In 2011, Marco Pelosi, a great Peruvian gynecologist who has developed his career in the United States, held the first congress of cosmetogynecology with an important attendance. One of his disciples, Dr. Alexander Bader, from Greece, who is also a disciple of Matlock creates, a few years later, the *European Society of Aesthetic Gynecology* that brings together hundreds of cosmetogynecologists every year in different cities of Europe.

Among the most relevant advances of labiaplasty is the fact that it stopped being a surgery for extreme cases practiced with certain disdain by the resident at the end of the surgical program in the morning of the public hospital or university after the operations considered important, to become part of the usual practice of aesthetic gynecology and—why not to say it—functional gynecology. In the last decade, the number of courses and congresses of the specialty in all continents is countless, and within these courses, labiaplasty and female genital aesthetics are a fundamental chapter.

It is not yet defined with certainty the advantages of the cutting instrument, whether it is laser, radiofrequency, or simple scissors and/or scalpel, but it is very clear that, despite the furious opposition of feminist groups and certain medical associations, especially American, they have not managed to prevent thousands (yes, thousands) of women from voluntarily undergoing a labiaplasty every year.

The accusations of FGM, overdiagnosis of hypertrophy, and surgical indication are to underestimate the intelligence of those women who voluntarily choose a cosmetic gynecologist and request his services.

The great last step is perfection of the surgical technique until there are no more doubts about which is the best and with less complications; discussion that exceeds this chapter of the book, but on the other hand, to consolidate this surgery as an absolutely ambulatory procedure and that, in my personal case, following the experience of great cosmetogynecologists such as Michael Goodman and Red Alinsod, I have almost totally turned to local anesthesia. At the time of writing this chapter, I no longer perform a single labiaplasty of the labia majora or labia minora under general or regional anesthesia; all are performed under local anesthesia. The exception is in patients where another surgery requiring major anesthesia must be performed, such as a hysterectomy and/or concomitant urinary incontinence correction.

Since I started performing labiaplasty on a regular basis, I have performed over a thousand cases, and it is one of the surgeries that has given me the most professional satisfaction, due to the very high degree of satisfied patients and the very low rate of complications. The cases of women who have carried the burden of having hypertrophic labia minora that have hindered and sometimes prevented them from having an acceptable sexual life are—in my experience—innumerable. The cry of relief after surgery that I have seen in many of my patients when they know that their burden is over continues to this day to thrill me. In reality and as I say in many presentations, cosmetic gynecology surgeries were not invented by cosmetogynecologists; they just did something that women were waiting for.

References

1. The Bible, Book of Genesis, Chapter 17.
2. Gruenbaum E. The female circumcision controversy. University of Pennsylvania Press; 2001.
3. Genital reconstructive surgery after female genital mutilation. Obstet Gynecol Int J. 2016;4(6).
4. Jaeger L. Obstetrics & Gynecology Sep 7, 2018.
5. Gynaecology. Vol 4. Latin translation of the treatise Gynaeciorum. Soranu of Ephesus.
6. Sixteen Books on Medicine. Aetios of Amida, 4th century.
7. News: Francis Adams (1796–1861). Nature. 1942;150(5):286–7.
8. Traité des Maladies des Femmes Grosses. Francois Mauriceau. 17th century.
9. Rouzier R, Louis-Sylvestre C, Paniel BJ, Haddad B. Hypertrophy of the labia minora: experience with 163 reductions. Am J Obstet Gynecol. 2000;182:35–40. "Labia minora are considered hypertrophic when the maximal distance between base and edge is >4 cm". (p. 35)
10. Braun V. In search of (better) sexual pleasure: female genital "cosmetic" surgery. Sexualities. 2005;8(4):407–24. "A lot of women bring in Playboy, show me pictures of vaginas and say: 'I want to look like this'".
11. J. Pardo, V. Solà, P. Ricci, E. Guilloff. Laser labioplasty of labia minora. Int J Gynecol Obstet. 2006;93:38–43.

Chapter 3
Topographical Anatomy

Pablo Gonzalez-Isaza

Introduction

Since our training in medical school, we may have seen and studied the same illustrations in different texts and atlases (Fig. 3.1), where the anatomy of the vulva is shown in a very basic way, for example, clitoral hood, clitoris, mons Venus, labia majora, labia minora, vestibule, and perineum, sometimes the frenulum of the clitoral hood is mentioned.

I consider that the anatomy of the vulva should be reviewed in a deeper way; we should talk about anatomical variants, particularities of the frenulum, aberrant insertions, as well as the innervation and vascularization, which together should be widely known at the time of performing a labiaplasty.

Now, I will describe the proposal of "topographic labiaplasty" (Fig. 3.2a, b), which is very useful when performing a labiaplasty; this concept arises from the need to identify not only anatomical landmarks but also to establish safe margins, to perform a labiaplasty in a reproducible and safe way.

P. Gonzalez-Isaza (✉)
Obstetrics and Gynecology Urogynecology Minimally Invasive Surgery Functional Cosmetic and Regenerative Gynecology, Hospital Universitario San Jorge/Liga contra el Cancer, Pereira, Madrid, Spain

© The Author(s), under exclusive license to Springer Nature Switzerland AG 2023
P. Gonzalez-Isaza, R. Sánchez-Borrego (eds.), *Topographic Labiaplasty*, https://doi.org/10.1007/978-3-031-15048-7_3

11

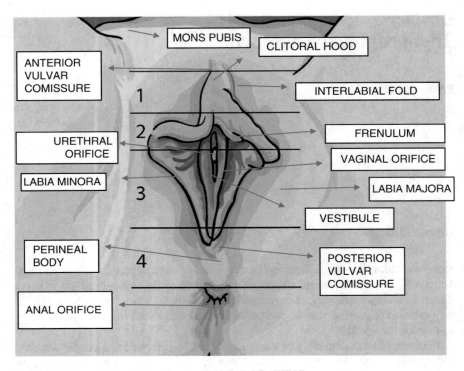

Fig. 3.1 Basic anatomy of the vulva. (PERSONAL DRAWING)

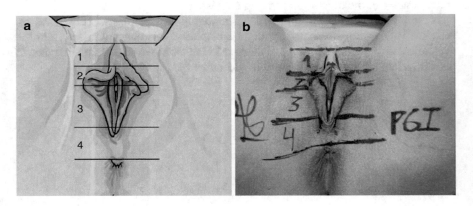

Fig. 3.2 (**a, b**) Anatomical zones

Anatomical Zones Fig. 3.2a, b

Zone 1
- Upper limit: anterior vulvar commissure
- Lower limit: apex (foreskin) of the clitoral hood

Zone 2
- Upper limit: apex of the clitoral hood (foreskin)
- Lower limit: insertion of the frenulum of the clitoral hood at the level of the labia minora

Zone 3
- Upper limit: cephalic insertion of the labium minora
- Inferior limit: caudal insertion of the labium minora

Zone 4
- Upper limit: base of the hymenal ring
- Lower limit: anal vertex

Each anatomical area has an anatomical repair called a safety zone.

- **Zone 1** (interlabial fold)
- **Zone 2** (frenulum/insertion complex)
- **Zone 3** (insertion base of the labia minora)
- **Zone 4** (distance from the perineal body at the level of the fourchette)

The main objectives of a topographic labiaplasty are:

- Identify safety landmarks

  – Anterior and posterior commissure location
  – Interlabial fold
  – Labia Minora-frenulum relationship
  – Perineal body height

- Approach all the components of labia minora hypertrophy

  – Labia minora
  – Clitoral hood-frenulum complex
  – Anatomical variants

      Horizontal plane (bifurcations duplications accessory folds)
      Vertical plane (ptosis or elongation of the clitoral hood)
      Excess skin at the level of posterior vulvar commissure

- Frenulum and its insertion preservation
- Interlabial fold preservation
- Preservation of anatomy and function
- To have as a final result cosmetically invisible wound
- Decrease the possibility of complications and poor aesthetic results

Moving forward with the concept, it is important to understand the anatomical particularities and aberrant insertions of the different structures.

Clitoral Hood Frenulum

Ostrzenski and collaborators [1] in their most recent research have found different anatomical definitions of this structure, such as "anterior bifurcation of the labium minora" or "inferior branch of the labium minora that inserts on the posterior surface of the glans of the clitoris." These concepts were taken from traditional books of anatomy even written by Graaf between 1668 and 1672.

For many years of performing labiaplasty, my biggest concern has always been this anatomical structure and its functions related to sexuality, specifically; it serves as a support and stabilization mechanism for the clitoral glans, connecting it to the apical portion of the labia minora, so that at the time of penetration a traction vector is generated from the perineum through the labia minora to the glans and clitoral hood [2].

It is not only its function but also the great number of anatomical variants (Fig. 3.3) that we can find around this structure when performing a labiaplasty, which is why I have decided to call it the "frenulum/insertion complex (Figs. 3.4, 3.5, and 3.6)."

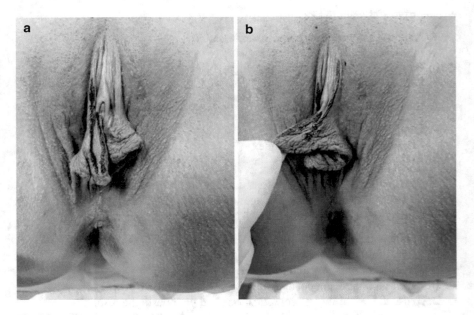

Fig. 3.3 (**a, b**) Aberrant distal insertion

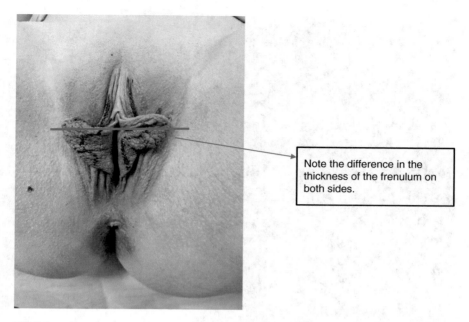

Note the difference in the thickness of the frenulum on both sides.

Fig. 3.4 Differences in the thickness of the frenulum: this is related to the amount of dartos fascia present in this structure

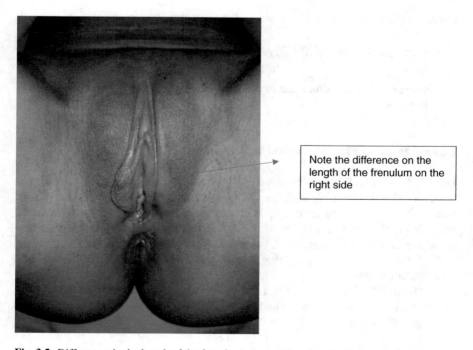

Note the difference on the length of the frenulum on the right side

Fig. 3.5 Differences in the length of the frenulum are considered anatomical particularities

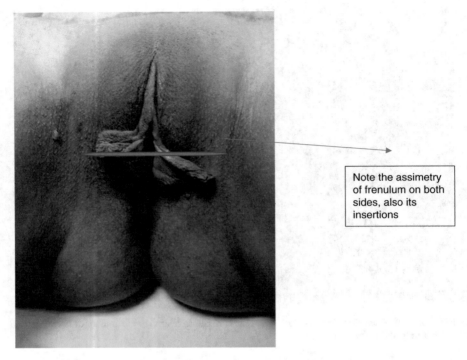

Note the assimetry of frenulum on both sides, also its insertions

Fig. 3.6 Asymmetric insertion of the frenulum at the apex of the labia minora

Aberrant Insertion of the Frenulum of the Clitoris

In this scenario the frenulum can be inserted on one side more distal compared to the other side.

Clitoral Hood and Its Anatomical Variants

One of the great fears when performing a labiaplasty is the approach to the clitoral hood, due to its relationship with the clitoris and sensitivity; in my experience, more than 80% of labiaplasty cases require a complementary approach to the clitoral hood, in order to offer a better aesthetic and functional result; the majority of secondary or revision labiaplasties are related to the omission to address this structure initially [3], that is, why I am going to carefully describe this fascinating topic of anatomical variants.

Hunter in 2015 is perhaps the first author who tries to describe in an orderly manner the anatomical variants at the level of the clitoral hood, basically describing two major groups (Table 3.1).

Table 3.1 Differences between a bifurcation and a duplication

Characteristics	Bifurcation	Duplication
Origin	Anterior vulvar commissure	Lateral and medial to the central portion of clitoral hood
Insertion	Frenulum, labia, perineal body	Frenulum lateral portion of labia minora, interlabial fold perineal body
Laterality	Unilateral, bilateral	Unilateral-bilateral
Observations	In some cases trifurcations are possible	In some cases, triplications and more accessory folds are possible

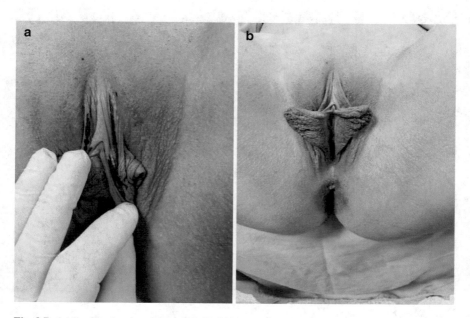

Fig. 3.7 (**a**) Duplication (caudal origin). (**b**) Bifurcation (cephalad origin)

(a) Anatomical variants in the vertical plane, which correspond to either ptosis or elongation of the clitoral hood and (b) Anatomical variants in the horizontal plane, which correspond to accessory folds parallel and lateral to the central portion of the clitoral hood, can be unilateral, bilateral, multiple, and asymmetrical [4].

Additionally, I have found bifurcations and even triplications of the clitoral hood (Figs. 3.7a, b, 3.8a, b, 3.9a, b, and 3.10) which start from its origin at the anterior vulvar commissure, and may insert either into the hood itself more distally or even into the labium minora and on rare occasions into the perineum or base of insertion of the labium Table 3.1. Such personal findings have not been previously described in the literature.

In some cases, there is also the possibility to find excess skin at the level of posterior vulvar commissure (Fig. 3.11).

Note in both sides a bifurcation, and its aberrant insertion in the lateral side of labia minora

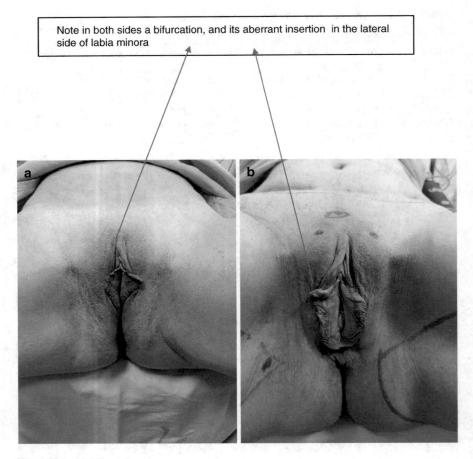

Fig. 3.8 (**a, b**) Bifurcation

Continuing with the anatomical variants in the clitoral hood, I have decided to describe an anomaly that I have frequently encountered, a fenestration of the clitoral hood (Fig. 3.12) and has also not been described in the literature, with some frequency, when approaching the clitoral hood, reviewing the literature has not been able to find this type of anatomical variant. However, the group of Brodie and collaborators found marked anatomical differences of the clitoral hood even from puberty [5]; from the morphological point of view, this feature may be related to the thickness of the dartos fascia.

Note in both sides, a duplication of clitoral hood with its aberrant insertion at the apex of right labia minora

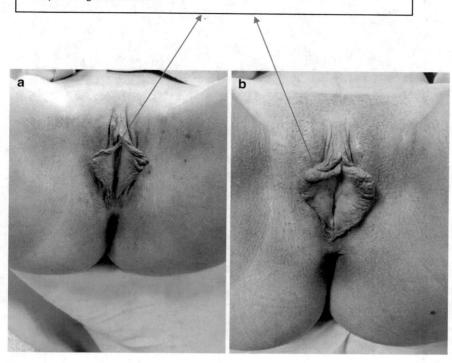

Fig. 3.9 (**a, b**) Duplication

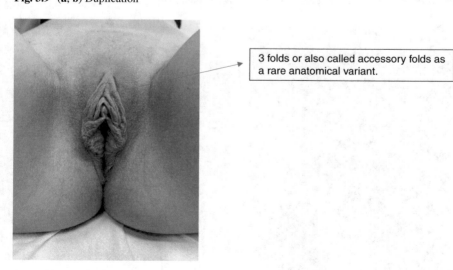

3 folds or also called accessory folds as a rare anatomical variant.

Fig. 3.10 Triplication

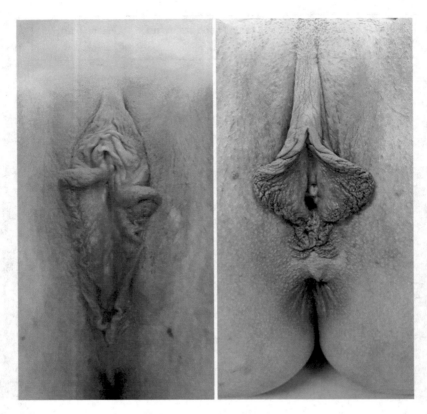

Fig. 3.11 Excess skin at the level of posterior vulvar commissure

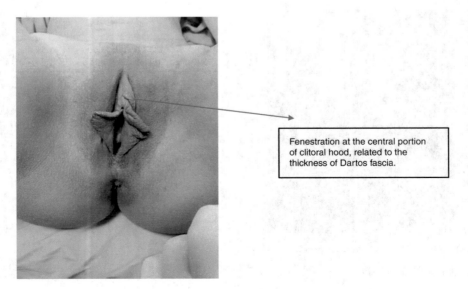

Fenestration at the central portion of clitoral hood, related to the thickness of Dartos fascia.

Fig. 3.12 Fenestrations at the level of the clitoral hood

References

1. Ostrzenski A. The clitoral infrafrenulum fascial bundle: the anatomy and histology. Clin Anat. 2018;31(6):907–12. https://doi.org/10.1002/ca.23215.
2. Rock JA, Jones HW, editors. Te Linde's operative gynecology. 11th ed. Philadelphia, PA: Wolters Kluwer; 2015. p. 93–4.
3. Hunter JG. Labia minora, labia majora, and clitoral hood alteration: experience-based recommendations. Aesthet Surg J. 2016;36(1):71–9. https://doi.org/10.1093/asj/sjv092.
4. Hunter JG. Commentary on: Postoperative clitoral hood deformity after labiaplasty. Aesthet Surg J. 2013;33(7):1037–8.
5. Brodie KE, Grantham EC, Huguelet PS, Caldwell BT, Westfall NJ, Wilcox DT. Study of clitoral hood anatomy in the pediatric population. J Pediatr Urol. 2016;12(3):177.e1–177.e1775. https://doi.org/10.1016/j.jpurol.2015.12.006.

Chapter 4
Classification of Labia Minora Hypertrophy

Pablo Gonzalez-Isaza

Introduction

The anatomical variability of the components of the vulva is very wide, which is why I have considered it to be very important to review the classifications available in the literature. Usually, the common denominator is to measure the length of labia minora in centimeters from the lateral aspect of the labia to the Haarts line from the most prominent area (Fig. 4.1).

Lloyd and colleagues [1] measured the labia minora in a group of 50 women between 18 and 50 years of age (mean 35.6), premenopausal patients of different ethnicities in the gynecology department of the London hospital, all reported a length between 20 and 100 mm (mean, 60.6; standard deviation, 17.2), while the width was between 7 and 50 mm (mean, 21.8; standard deviation, 9.4), while the width was between 7 and 50 mm (mean, 21.8; standard deviation, 9.4). The size was independent of age, parity, ethnicity, use of hormonal drugs, and history of sexual activity.

Currently there is a debate between pediatricians, plastic surgeons, and gynecologists regarding the classification of labia minora hypertrophy [2]. One of the first authors in the literature who proposed a measure to consider the labia minora hypertrophic was Friedrich, who in his publication considered a size greater than 50 mm in length [3]. On the other hand, Laufer and Munhoz considered hypertrophic labia minora if they exceeded a length of 30–40 mm [4, 5]. Hodgkinson, in his publication, also considered hypertrophic labia minora if these measure more than 5 cm [6] (Table 4.1).

P. Gonzalez-Isaza (✉)
Obstetrics and Gynecology Urogynecology Minimally Invasive Surgery Functional Cosmetic and Regenerative Gynecology, Hospital Universitario San Jorge/Liga contra el Cancer, Pereira, Madrid, Spain

P. Gonzalez-Isaza, R. Sánchez-Borrego (eds.), *Topographic Labiaplasty*,
https://doi.org/10.1007/978-3-031-15048-7_4

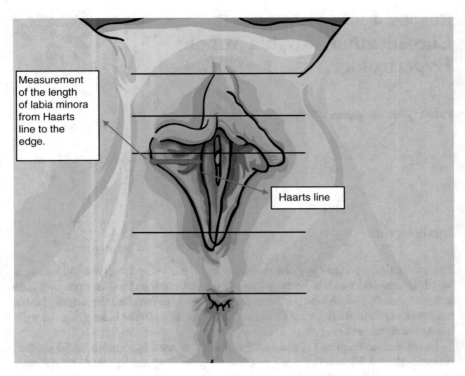

Measurement of the length of labia minora from Haarts line to the edge.

Haarts line

Fig. 4.1 Labia minora length measurement explanation. (Personal Drawing)

Table 4.1 Different classifications of labia minora hypertrophy

Classification	Author	Characteristics	Advantages/disadvantages	Disadvantages
Radmann	Radmann 1963	> 5 cm	Length	No other components
Fiedrich	Friedrich 1983	>5 cm	Length	No other components
Talita Franco	Yelda Felicio 1992 Francia	>6 cm	Length	No other components
Alter	Alter 1995	Simetria	Evaluation of other components	NA
Pardo/Ricci/ Sola	1998	Severidad	Severity is a subjective interpretation	NA
Rouzzieer	2000	>4 cm	Length	No other components
Saba Motakef	2015	>4 cm	Considers indirectly anatomical variants	No other components
Colaneri	2017	>5 cm	Classified with grades 0, 1, 2, 3 considers labia minora and clitoral hood as independent units	

There are several classifications for the approach of labia minora hypertrophy; the common denominator is the measurement of the size in centimeters; when reviewing them thoroughly I found, for example, the group of Dr. Saba Motakef divides it into three degrees according to the length in cm from the interlabial fold to the most distal portion of the lip as follows: Saba Motakef group divides it in three grades according to the length in cm from the interlabial fold to the most distal portion of the labia as follows: grade I (0–2 cm), grade II (2–4 cm), and grade III (greater than 4 cm). Additionally the author adds a letter "A" in case of asymmetry and a letter "C" in case of compromise of the clitoral hood, omitting other components of the vulva involved in the hypertrophy of the labia minora [7].

Chang and collaborators proposed a new classification system "snip and clip" that consists of describing hypertrophy according to its anatomical location as follows:

- Class 1: less than 2 cm "moderate," protrusion of the labia minora beyond the posterior vulvar commissure, may be visible, but without exceeding the labia majora
- Class 2: greater than 2 cm, protrusion of the labia minora, beyond the posterior vulvar commissure, and with extension to the labia majora
- Class 3: may include class 2, tissue that protrudes above the clitoris in a separate area
- Class 4: may include class 2 or 3, protrusion of tissue beyond the perineal body and anus [8]

Regarding severity, it is important to emphasize that from the ethical point of view it is difficult to put adjectives to this clinical condition as mild, moderate, or severe, since a small hypertrophy for a patient can be severe and a large hypertrophy for a patient may not be bothersome at all; for this reason I believe that the degree of severity is not a component that should be taken into account inside a classification of labia minora hypertrophy, in the same way the group of Dr. Pardo and colleagues catalog some types of hypertrophy in their series, as mild, moderate, or severe, which I find difficult to interpret, taking into account the great anatomical variability present in the vulva [9].

Smarrito and collaborators made a 9-year-follow-up in more than 100 patients describing basically three types of labia minora hypertrophy as follows:

- Type I: excess skin located in the anterior third without involvement in other areas, "flag shape."
- Type II: excess skin at the level of the anterior and middle third "oblique shape."
- Type III: excess skin in the posterior third [10] (Fig. 4.2).

Returning to the common denominator (length in centimeters), the group of Talita and Franco in 1993 described their classification in four grades as follows:

- **I Less than 2 cm**
- **II from 2 to 4 cm**
- **III from 4 to 6 cm**
- **IV larger than 6 cm**

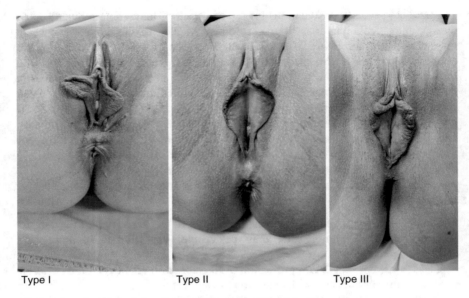

Type I   Type II   Type III

Fig. 4.2 Interpretation of classification of Smarrito and collaborators

However, when a more extensive search was made, it was found that this classification is originally described by a French author Yhelda Felicio in 1992 and was erroneously assigned to Talita-Franco [11].

Continuing with the extensive search of classifications, we find one more described by Dr. Cunha and collaborators; in this classification the author tries to describe the anatomical variants that are directed from the clitoral hood or the posterior vulvar commissure [12] (Figs. 4.3, 4.4, and 4.5).

With all the previous classifications, there has been an immense interest on the part of the authors to express their own or their group's vision about labia minora hypertrophy and what in their opinion could be a classification system, which is why I consider them to be basic classifications and not very reproducible, from the point of view of surgical planning techniques, which is why since 2015, I had the idea of proposing a classification that adequately described all the components involved in labia minora hypertrophy, such as the clitoral hood, the labia minora, and the posterior vulvar commissure (Fig. 4.6), additionally, to evaluate and classify the symmetry, since these characteristics are very important when planning a proper surgical technique for a labiaplasty. Finally, after several months of work I was able to publish it [1, 13]:

It consists of three parts:

1. **Length (centimeters)**

    I Less than 2 cm
    II 2–4 cm
    III 4–6 cm
    IV larger than 6 cm

Fig. 4.3 Interpretation of classification of Cunha type I

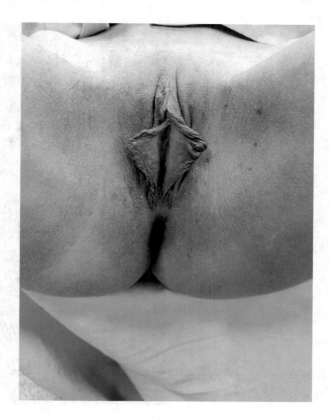

2. **Location**

   (A) in those hypertrophies that have a predominantly anterior involvement.
   (B) in those hypertrophies that have a central predominant involvement.
   (C) in those hypertrophies that have a predominantly generalized involvement.

3. **Symmetry**

   (S) in symmetric hypertrophies.
   (A) in asymmetric hypertrophies.

In such a way that in this classification, the three most important aspects in a labia minora hypertrophy, such as the length, the anatomical area involved, and the symmetry, I consider when planning the best surgical technique that suits the anatomy of the patients, in order to obtain better results, from the aesthetic, functional, and sexual point of view.

As an example, I present the following clinical case that will facilitate the understanding of this classification, and therefore its application will be easier.

Fig. 4.4 Interpretation of classification of Cunha type II

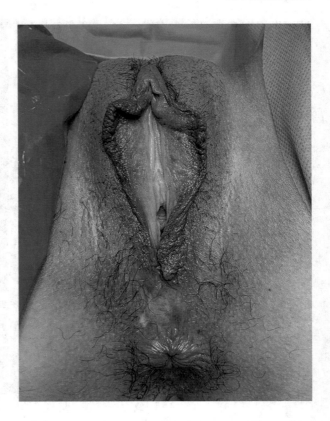

Twenty-five-year-old patient with excess tissue at the level of the labia minora distributed toward the clitoral hood of the labia proper, greater than 6 cm predominantly on the right side and at the level of the posterior vulvar commissure.

It can be interpreted as:

- **Hypertrophy of labia minora: IV-C-A** (Fig. 4.7).
  where

    IV—is the size in centimeters
    C—is the generalized compromise
    A—asymmetry due to predominance on the right side

Additionally, the presence of anatomical variants and their location in the horizontal plane can be added to the clinical assessment, e.g., duplications, bifurcations, and trifurcations of the clitoral hood, and in the vertical plane, ptosis and elongation of the clitoral hood.

Work is currently underway to validate the classification at an international level.

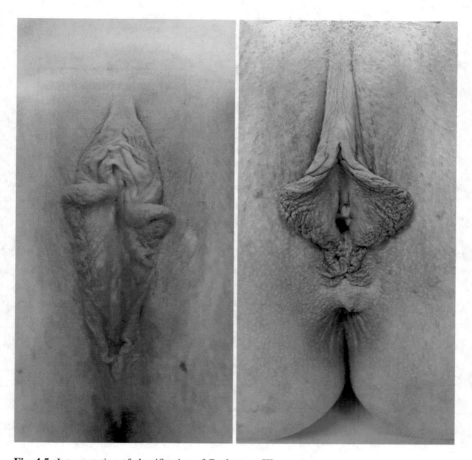

Fig. 4.5 Interpretation of classification of Cunha type III

TYPE OF HYPERTROPHY	LOCALIZATION	SIMETRY
I < 2 CMS	A ANTERIOR	SYMETRIC
II 2-4 CMS	B CENTRAL	ASYMETRIC
III 4-6 CMS	C GENERALIZED	
IV > 6 CMS		

Fig. 4.6 Gonzalez classification diagram

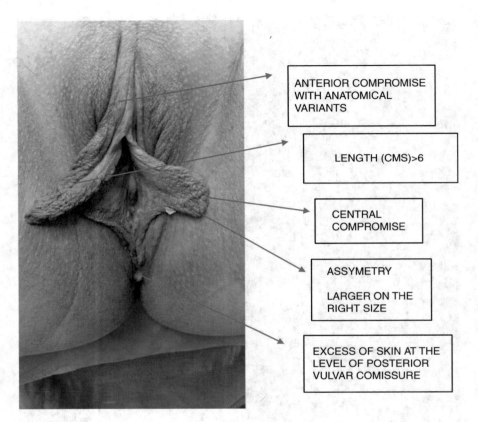

Fig. 4.7 Example of Gonzalez classification IV-C-A

Finally, the group of Colaneri and collaborators in Brazil consider with their experience of more than 400 labiaplasties that something is missing in my classification, and I understand that they refer to the presence of anatomical variants, and degrees of labia minora hypertrophy are considered according to the length of the labia measured in centimeters, from Haarts line to the lateral aspect of the labia (Fig. 4.8) [14].

As I mentioned before, I consider important not only the clinical validation of all these classifications but also their easy applicability and usefulness in the context of surgical planning.

O	1cms	A.Labia minora
1	2 cms	B.Clitoral Hood
2	3 cms	
3	4 cms	

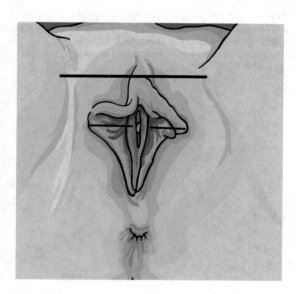

Fig. 4.8 Interpretation of classification from Colanery et al.

References

1. Lloyd J, Crouch NS, Minto CL, Liao LM, Creighton SM. Female genital appearance: "normality" unfolds. BJOG. 2005;112:643–6.
2. Hailparn TR. What is a girl to do?: the problem of adolescent labial hypertrophy. Obstet Gynecol. 2014;123(Suppl 1):124S–5S.
3. Friedrich EG. Vulvar disease. 2nd ed. Philadelphia: Saunders; 1983.
4. Laufer MR, Galvin WJ. Labia hypertrophy: a new surgical approach. Adolesc Pediatr Gynecol. 1995;8:39–41.
5. Munhoz AM, Filassi JR, Ricci MD, Aldrighi C, Correia LD, Aldrighi JM, et al. Aesthetic labia minora reduction with inferior Wedge resection and superior pedicle flap reconstruction. Plast Reconstr Surg. 2006;118:1237–47. discussion 1248–50
6. Hodgkinson DJ, Hait G. Aesthetic vaginal labioplasty. Plast Reconstr Surg. 1984;74(3):414–6.
7. Motakef S, Rodriguez-Feliz J, Ingargiola MJ, Chung MT, Patel A. Reply: Vaginal labiaplasty: current practices and a simplified classification system for labial protrusion. Plast Reconstr Surg. 2015;136(5):706e–7e. https://doi.org/10.1097/PRS.0000000000001666.
8. Chang P, Salisbury MA, Narsete T, Buckspan R, Derrick D, Ersek RA. Vaginal labiaplasty: defense of the simple "clip and snip" and a new classification system. Aesthet Plast Surg. 2013;37(5):887–91. https://doi.org/10.1007/s00266-013-0150-0.

9. Pardo J, Solà V, Ricci P, Guilloff E. Laser labioplasty of labia minora. Int J Gynaecol Obstet. 2006;93(1):38–43. https://doi.org/10.1016/j.ijgo.2006.01.002.
10. Smarrito S. Classification of labia minora hypertrophy: a retrospective study of 100 patient cases. JPRAS Open. 2017;13:81–91.
11. Felicio Y. Chirurgie intime. Rev Chir Esth Lang Franc. 1992;27(67):37–43.
12. Cunha FI, Silva LM, Costa LA, Vasconcelos FRP, Amaral GT. Nymphoplatia: classification and technical refinements. Rev Bras Cir Plást. 2011;26(3):507–11.
13. Colaneri AG d F. Nova classificação para hipertrofia dos pequenos lábios vaginais e correlação com as técnicas cirúrgicas indicadas/New classification of hypertrophy of the labia minora and correlation with indicated surgical techniques. Rev Bras Cir Plást. 2018;33(1):64–73.
14. Gonzalez P. Labia minora hypertrophy classification consideration of a multiple component approach. Surg Tech Int. 2015;27:191–4.

Chapter 5
Labia Minora Labiaplasty: Surgical Techniques

Juan José Escribano Tórtola and Gloria Rodea Gaspar

Introduction

The surgical reduction of the labia minora as a treatment for their hypertrophy is called labiaplasty (LP). The etiology of the increase in size of the labia minora is unknown, being related to various causes, congenital, hormonal, trauma, or repeated infections, although it is important to specify the concept, from our point of view, that there are multiple variants of "normality" of the vulva and therefore should not make pathological what really is not. Discouraging the concept of normal or abnormal in the external genitalia is one of the objectives that any professional whose aim will be to surgically address the vulva from a comprehensive point of view, in those patients that for multiple reasons related to their labia minora see their quality of life affected [1–5].

The lack of a clear definition of labia minora hypertrophy and the existence of multiple classifications make it difficult to establish clear and common criteria for performing the technique. As a general rule, it is established as protrusion beyond the vulvar labia majora and can generally be accompanied by hypertrophy of the clitoral hood [6, 7].

J. J. E. Tórtola (✉)
Department of Obstetrics and Gynecology, Severo Ochoa University Hospital, Madrid, Spain

Unit of Regenerative, Functional and Aesthetic Gynecology, Laser Medical Institute, Madrid, Spain

G. R. Gaspar
Unit of Regenerative, Functional and Aesthetic Gynecology, Laser Medical Institute, Madrid, Spain

Unit of Gynecology, Gran Vía Clinic, Madrid, Spain

© The Author(s), under exclusive license to Springer Nature Switzerland AG 2023
P. Gonzalez-Isaza, R. Sánchez-Borrego (eds.), *Topographic Labiaplasty*, https://doi.org/10.1007/978-3-031-15048-7_5

The demand for this type of surgery has been increasing in recent years. Data from the American Society of Aesthetic Plastic Surgeons in 2017 reports an increase of 217.2% since 2012 [3].

The reasons why patients request labiaplasty are divided into aesthetic (generally), functional, and/or mixed reasons. The perception of the "abnormal" appearance of the labia minora, which affects self-esteem, is influenced by sociocultural reasons, the media, family environment, sexual partners, etc. [8–11]. The detailed and individualized clinical history is vital to rule out possible psychosexological affectations (consider the presence of dysmorphophobic syndrome), which interfere in this perception, and to determine what are the real expectations of the patient and what we intend to achieve with surgery [12, 13].

Up to 11 different techniques have been described for performing a labiaplasty. The main objective of the surgery is that the patient in standing position is observed minimal or no protrusion of the labia minora over the labia majora. Of all the techniques, linear excision (edge or trim) and wedge excision are the most commonly performed, followed by Z-plasty and the de-epithelialization technique, although there is no technique defined as gold standard in the literature reviewed [1–3]. The complication rates of this surgery are low, 2–5%, and the degree of satisfaction obtained by patients is over 90% [3].

The limitations we found to perform a systematic review of the subject are the lack of uniformity of inclusion criteria based primarily on the lack of a universal classification [6, 7, 14, 15], the small sample size of the published studies, and the lack of studies with adequate design that mean the number of minor and major complications, the long-term follow-up period, and the degree of satisfaction obtained with validated questionnaires [1]. The surgical procedure to be performed should be based on the anatomy of the vulva, the realistic expectations, and goals of the patient [16–19].

In this chapter we will deal with the techniques described on the basis of the existing scientific support, with the aim of facilitating surgeons the most appropriate choice for each case.

Surgical Techniques

In relation to the origin of the surgical techniques, we will mention some relevant moments. Martincik and Malinovsky in 1971 described the resection of a triangle of tissue in the posterior part of the labia minora with suture of both margins [20]. In 1976, Radman, published two cases of labia minora hypertrophy in which he performed a labiaplasty using the linear resection technique. This was the first time the procedure was performed under medical indication [21]. The first article published in an American journal referring to labiaplasty was in 1978. Honoré et al. presented two cases of bilateral elongation of the labia minora of the vulva in which a surgical resection was performed, due to the discomfort of the patients [22]. Hodgkinson and Hait, in 1984, performed the direct technique for the first time with a description of plastic surgery and for aesthetic purposes, referring for the first time to the importance of the influence of the media and the culture of the image in the perception of the "ideal" vulva [23].

An important change in the approach to labia minora hypertrophy was in 1998, when Alter described a new surgical technique, consisting of a wedge resection, changing the perspectives of the procedures performed to date, and serving as a model for successive modifications that would be made by other authors, from that moment on [24].

The main objective of any surgical technique is to preserve as much of the anatomy as possible, maintaining functionality with the best possible aesthetic result. Several systematic review articles on the techniques have been reported to date.

Motakef et al. in 2015 presented the results of the analysis of a selection of 19 articles from 247 publications. They evaluated 16 retrospective studies and 3 clinical cases and analyzed, based on their classification of the degree of labial hypertrophy, 7 surgical techniques including the one performed by laser (direct excision, de-epithelialization, wedge, W-technique, composite technique, Z-plasty, and laser), finding a 94–100% satisfaction rate and a very low rate of complications, the most frequent being suture dehiscence with 4.7%.They concluded that labiaplasty is a safe procedure with a high rate of satisfaction, recommending randomized studies with unified criteria for the classification of hypertrophy, to compare some techniques with others and obtain results that allow to establish the best option [25, 26].

In the same year, Oranges et al. published a review of eight techniques (composite labiaplasty, wedge, de-epithelialization, direct excision, laser, custom flask, W-technique, and fenestrated technique with flap transposition). Sixty-four articles were initially identified and 38 studies, 29 retrospective, and 9 case reports were selected. The satisfaction rate exceeded 90%, and a 6.7% complication rate was reported. The authors concluded that the eight techniques analyzed presented good results with low morbidity and a high degree of patient satisfaction [2].

Özer et al., in 2018 [1], published a review of labiaplasty techniques also addressing patients' motivations toward such surgery and the ethical considerations surrounding it. They analyzed 11 described techniques of labiaplasty with the outcomes and complications of each. They divided them into three groups (edge resection or direct linear resection, wedge resection, and central resection), depending on the area and shape of the incision and the labial tissue to be preserved (Figs. 5.1, 5.2, 5.3, 5.4, 5.5, and 5.6).

The edge or trim technique [27] consists in the resection of the excess of the hypertrophic labia and its edge and can be performed by a linear incision (Fig. 5.1a), which follows the curvature of the lip [28], by an elongated "S"-shaped incision or "S lazy-lazy" (Fig. 5.1b) [29] which aims to lengthen the scar and thus reduce the tension, or by a W-shaped incision [30], performed alternatively on the inner and outer face of the lip with the intention of adjusting the scarring more easily (Fig. 5.1c). A variant of the latter is the Z-plasty technique (Fig. 5.3), widely used in plastic surgery with the intention of reducing the length of the scar [2]. It is essential in this type of surgery to preserve Hart's line on the inner side of labia minora,

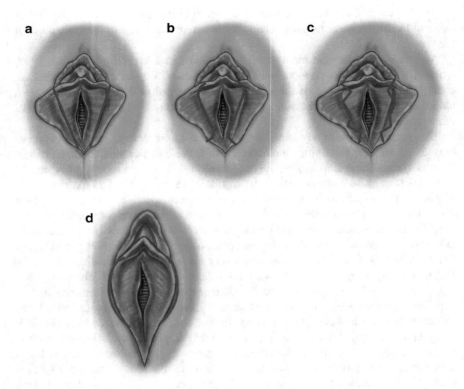

Fig. 5.1 (**a–c**) Preoperative linear resection techniques. (**d**) Postoperative linear resection technique

leaving at least 0.5–1 cm as safe margins outside of it, in order to perform an amputation of the labia minora [3].

The wedge resection technique (wedge resection), together with the linear technique, is the most frequently used of all. It presents several modifications with the aim of improving the aesthetic results (preserving the shape and the border of the labia minora) and functional, considering the most affected labial area with hypertrophy (classification used) [7], and its vascularization (central, superior, and inferior labial artery), to design the central wedge, anterior, or posterior [1, 3]. The central wedge described by Alter [24] and the rest of variants can be performed preserving the main vascularization [24, 30, 31] (Fig. 5.2). With the intention of reducing the length of the scar and avoiding retractions, Giraldo et al. perform a Z-plasty at 90° (Fig. 5.3) [32]. Another surgical variant (Fig. 5.4) is the performance of a posterior wedge using the technique performed by Rouzier and Kelishadi [33, 34] and the inferior wedge resection with reconstruction of the pedicle of the superior flap described by Munhoz [35]. The third group of techniques are those that approach the labia minora with the aim of preserving their original pigmentation, contour, and texture by means of de-epithelialization. This procedure described by

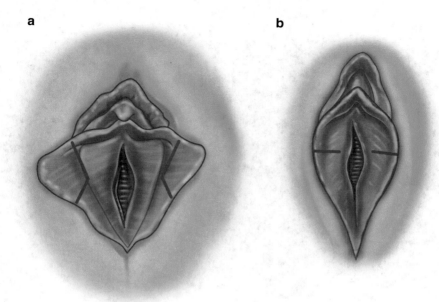

Fig. 5.2 Alter's central wedge (**a**) Pre-operative (**b**) Post-operative

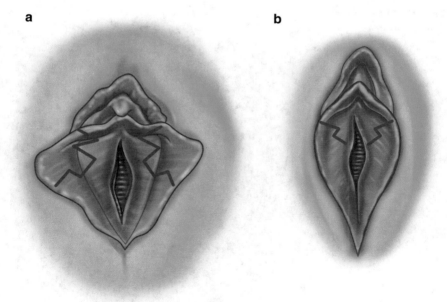

Fig. 5.3 Giraldo et al.'s Z-plasty (**a**) Preoperative (**b**) Postoperative

a

b

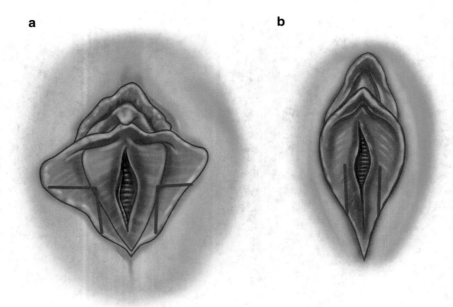

Fig. 5.4 Rouzier and Kelishadi's posterior wedge (**a**) Preoperative (**b**) Postoperative

Fig. 5.5 Ostrzenski et al.'s "cyclist's helmet"

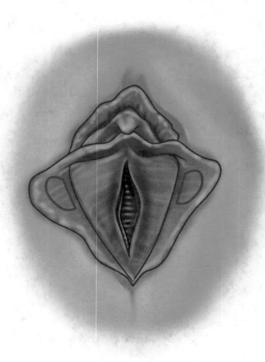

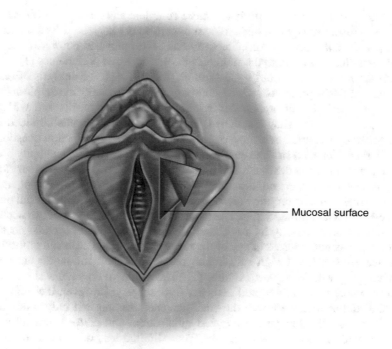

Mucosal surface

Fig. 5.6 Choi et al.'s de-epithelialization

Choi et al. consists of designing a central triangle on the inner and outer face of the labia minora and removing the epidermal tissue; unfortunately high rates of dehiscence are being reported inside the literature, and the technique is abandoned by many surgeons [36] (Figs. 5.5 and 5.6), and the fenestration technique, proposed by Ostrzenski et al. that removes the hypertrophic tissue by a design in the form of a "cyclist's helmet" [37].

The use of laser technology for excision of labia minora hypertrophic tissue has increased in recent years due to the beneficial properties of this type of energy. Pardo et al., in 2006 [38], and Smarrito, in 2014 [39], report a series of 55 and 231 cases operated with laser with effective and safe results. In 2018, Gonzalez et al. demonstrated histopathological results, in a comparative study of labiaplasty using different types of CO_2 laser-designed pulses, the benefits obtained by applying this form of energy [40].

When selecting a labiaplasty technique, it would be very useful to have certain criteria to guide us toward one technique or another. In this regard, Ellsworth et al. [41] published a decision algorithm that allows, based on the type of hypertrophy and the patient's request for maintenance of the labia minora edge, the linear technique, the wedge technique, or de-epithelialization. This algorithm is determined by Franco's initial classification, which in 2015 was modified by González et al., providing, from our point of view, a more complete and anatomical differentiation of the degrees and types of labia minora hypertrophy [1, 7]. However, no other system for selecting the type of labiaplasty has been published before; the technique chosen varies according to the surgeon's experiences and preferences [1].

In the review carried out by Özer et al., in 2018, [1], the analysis of results of several studies is presented, which show a great heterogeneity in sample size, in the follow-up period, with unadjusted criteria to define the results and with a poor degree of evidence. They concluded that, in general, the results obtained are not supported by scientific evidence, requiring standardized satisfaction questionnaires for their correct analysis. The complications reported are minor, generally bleeding, pain, hematoma, and dehiscence of the surgical wound, and there are four studies in this review in which are not described. Most complications resolved spontaneously. Major complications required revision surgery in four studies, and sexual problems were described in three studies. The most serious complication that can occur, labia minora amputation, with its associated physical, sexual, and psychological consequences, was not reported in any of the reviewed studies [1]. Eleven of the 16 studies analyzed reported high satisfaction rates throughout follow-up but were not evaluated by validated questionnaires [1]. The results of the review showed overall improvement in sensitivity and sexuality after surgery. However, the limitations of all the studies reviewed were the small sample size and that only a few of them reported complication rates, evaluated satisfaction, and performed a follow-up to assess medium- and long-term results. These limitations prevented us from obtaining validated conclusions, and we recommend the use of pre- and postsurgical questionnaires oriented to this type of surgery, such as the GAS, COPS, and COPS-L scales [13, 42–44].

As previously mentioned, of all the techniques described in the labiaplasty literature, the two most frequently used are the linear resection technique (edge or trim) and the wedge resection technique, with its central, inferior, and superior variants. We will describe each of them in brief.

Linear Resection Technique

It is the most frequently used technique, in its curved linear variant, with 52.7% [45], since most women who undergo labia minora reduction wish to eliminate the hyperpigmented border of the labia minora, maintaining the natural appearance they desire [46]. This type of surgery presents fewer complications related to wound healing but can sometimes lead to wound retraction pain and dyspareunia [15]. Healing, as in most techniques, usually progresses normally and usually goes unnoticed 6 months after surgery. Although they are usually performed with classic cutting instruments (scalpel, scissors, electrosurgical units, etc.), some advantages related to safety, efficacy, and functional and aesthetic results have been described in the literature when using laser and radiofrequency [38, 40, 47].

The surgical technique itself begins with the correct markings of the incision lines using a surgical pen, laterally and below the frenulum, (1–1.5 cm approximate safe margin), descending on the inner side up to the vulvar vestibule, always leaving Hart's line as an internal safety margin, to avoid excessive resection of labial tissue and scar retractions and amputation of labia minora. On the external side of the labia, the incision line, also circular in shape, will cover from the apex of the labia to the lower insertion, also leaving about 1.5 cm of safety distance to the interlabial fold, which is located between labia majora and labia minora. The surgical design in the contralateral labia will try to reproduce in a symmetrical way what was previously done in the first one, in cases of symmetrical hypertrophy, adapting in the best possible way in cases of asymmetrical hypertrophy, to achieve the best anatomical, functional, and aesthetic result possible. The aim is to be as much conservative as possible with the excision, although in this technique, there are variants depending on the amount of hypertrophic tissue to be excised [15] (Fig. 5.7).

The surgical incision is made following the marked lines, trying to place the cutting instrument as perpendicular to the tissue as possible, and in those cases in which there is a large volume of tissue to be removed due to the labial thickness, the incision can be angled in the central area of the labia to favor the adherence of the labial edges. We must be very meticulous when removing the possible "dog ears" that may appear as excess tissue lateral to the frenulum, frequently related to the

Fig. 5.7 Different incision
lines according to the
amount of hypertrophic
tissue to be removed

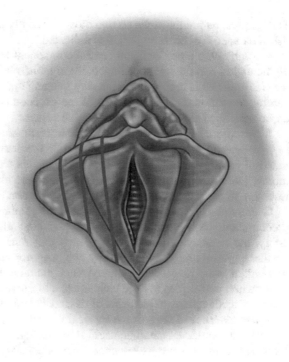

anatomical variants of the clitoral hood. Once adequate hemostasis has been carried out, closure of the surgical wound can be carried out in different ways depending on the authors; to date there is no standardized suture technique and/or type of suture material to be used in a systematic way [1–3, 25]. In general, a layered suture is carried out, with loose stitches, in the subcutaneous tissue with absorbable mono-filament 4 or 5-0.This type of suture persists longer than multifilament sutures, maintaining the adherence necessary for proper healing. For the last layer, loose stitches are usually used with multifilament absorbable sutures, generally fast-absorption polyglactine 4 or 5-0, which allow the edges to be brought closer together very effectively. Regardless of the types of sutures, stitches, and layers used and sutured, we must consider as basic rules of the technique to avoid dead spaces to prevent abscesses and hematomas, not to apply too much tension in the sutured area to avoid necrosis and suture the edges facing the planes correctly, to avoid including the skin in the subcutaneous area and prevent inclusion cysts. In general, it is recommended not to use continuous suture in the superficial layer to avoid the effects of protrusions in the labial border. Many surgeons perform an intradermal suture in the last layer to hide the suture line and improve the aesthetic appearance of the scar [1–3, 15, 47].

Wedge Resection Technique

This surgical technique is the second most frequently performed, according to published data, 36% of the time [45]. It is indicated in patients who present labia minora hypertrophy with a predominant central component and who wish to maintain the pigmentation and natural appearance of the labia minora edge. It allows to reduce the size of the labia in a proportional way, keeping their morphological structure and natural coloration. It is summarized in the excision of a wedge-shaped portion of tissue with an external base and an internal vertex.

A current surgical trend is to preserve the subcutaneous tissue of the labia minora to be removed (Fig. 5.8), in order to maintain the neurovascular bundle of the sub-mucosal territory. Some authors describe that this technique is more effective in thinner labia than in thicker ones. In summary, the idea it is to adapt the mucosal resection to give shape to the labia minora with great hypertrophy [1, 15].

Charalambous et al., in 2015, published the vascular anatomy of the labia minora, predominantly dependent on the internal pudendal artery. They presented a central artery, the most important, with a branch that runs along the anterior border, a smaller superior artery, and generally two posterior arteries [48]. It is important to be familiar with this vascular supply when planning the surgical technique, especially when performing wedge techniques and its variants as well as in the linear resection technique, to avoid areas of tissue ischemia with its corresponding necrosis and dehiscence of flaps or the surgical wound.

As for the surgical technique itself, it begins with a correct design of the incision lines by means of a surgical marker. The shape, size, and position of the incision

Fig. 5.8 Complete wedge resection technique with preservation of the neurovascular bundle [15]

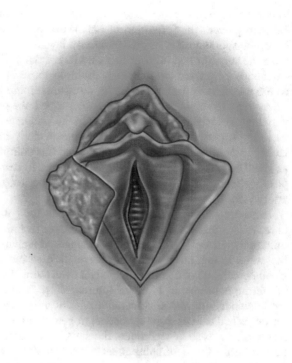

margins is of vital importance to achieve the expected results and avoid complications, which in this type of technique are also usually minor, highlighting for its importance the higher frequency of dehiscence of the suture line [1–3]. The design will be made on both labial sides, respecting a safety margin of 0.5 cm from the urethral meatus, on the inner side of the labia minora, to avoid possible alterations in the urinary flow related to abnormal scarring. In general, and depending on the type of labia minora hypertrophy, the wedge is designed as centrally as possible on the thickest component of the labia, and with the idea of preserving vascular supply in the rest of the labia, and also is kept as anterior as possible. Many authors prefer more anterior wedges for this reason [15, 48].

The incision can be made using the instruments described in the linear technique. In the case of using energy-based devices, those that cause the least lateral thermal damage and improve healing should be preferred. CO_2 laser has shown histopathological advantages over the rest [40]. Once the prominent portion of the labia has been resected, de-epithelializing as much as possible, especially in the case of thin labia, and hemostasis is achieved, the surgical wound is closed separately, both on the inner and outer side. The same reabsorbable sutures described above (5-0 monofilament) are used, emphasizing the importance of the first submucous suture line that joins the upper and lower flaps of the base of the wedge on both sides. It is a submucosal stitch, which can be of the mattress type, fairly approximated to be able to maintain the transverse suture line in surgical wound. In addition, this first stitch helps to prevent the formation of notches or protrusions in the apex of the flaps. Next, the submucosa is sutured in several layers and with loose stitches to approximate the superior and inferior flaps, on its medial side and lateral side. Finally, the cutaneous edges are sutured with multiple loose stitches, without tension, with resorbable sutures (monofilament or rapid absorption polydiaxone 5-0) [15, 49].

As in all the labiaplasty techniques described, the percentage of complications is very low, and most of them are minor. In the wedge technique, wound dehiscence is more important than in linear resection, especially in smokers, which is why the latter is recommended. The advice to avoid this complication is to make the wedge as small as possible to reduce the tension and to resect the tissue as anteriorly as possible (anterior wedge), in order to avoid the lesion of the central labia minora artery [15].

In summary, the current growing demand for genital aesthetic surgical procedures means that we must update the available techniques for the treatment of labia minora hypertrophy. To date, no gold standard technique has been described in the literature; in fact all of them are safe, with high rates of patient satisfaction and a small percentage of complications. Not even there is a standard criterion for the use of cutting instruments, types of sutures, shape, and suture material. Similarly, the recommendations and postoperative care of this surgery are not homogeneous. All the published studies show a great heterogeneity in relation to the number of patients analyzed, the type of technique, the satisfaction criteria, the number of complications described, and the subsequent control. To the extent that we want to implement a "gold standard" technique, which meets the objectives of achieving anatomical integrity as much as possible, the functionality of the genital area, and with the best aesthetic result, we must design high-level comparative studies, with validated questionnaires and long-term follow-up, which allow conclusions with a sufficient degree of scientific evidence [1–3, 14, 15, 25, 49].

References

1. Özer M, Mortimore I, Jansma EP, Mullender MG. Labiaplasty: motivation, techniques and ethics. Nat Rev Urol. 2018;15(3):175–89.
2. Orange CM, Sisti A, Giovanni S. Labia minora reduction techniques: a comprehensive literature review. Aesthet Surg J. 2015;35(4):419–31.
3. Willis RH, Wong CS, Patel BC. Labiaplasty labia minora reduction. StatPearls Publishing LLC; 2020. Last UpDate: February 10, 2020. Bookshelf ID: NBK448086. PMID: 28846226.
4. Hagisawa S, Arisaka O. Effect of excess estrogen on breast and external genitalia development in growth hormone deficiency. J Pediatr Adolesc Gynecol. 2012;25:61–3.
5. Elective female genital cosmetic surgery: ACOG Committee Opinion, Number 795. Obstet Gynecol. 2020;135(1):e36–42. https://doi.org/10.1097/AOG.0000000000003616.
6. Chang P, Salisbury MA, Narsete T, Buckspan R, Derrick D, Ersek RA. Vaginal labiaplasty: defense of the simple "clip and snip" and a new classification system. Aesthet Plast Surg. 2013;37:887–91.

7. Gonzalez PI. Classification of hypertrophy of labia minora: consideration of a multiple component approach. Surg Technol Int. 2015;27:191–4.
8. Miklos JR, Moore RD. Labiaplasty of the labia minora: patients' indications for pursuing surgery. J Sex Med. 2008;5:1492–5.
9. Zwier S. "What motivates her": motivations for considering labial reduction surgery as recounted on women's online communities and surgeons' websites. Sex Med. 2014;2:16–23.
10. Hamori CA. Aesthetic surgery of the female genitalia: labiaplasty and beyond. Plast Reconstr Surg. 2014;134:661–73.
11. Sorice SC, Li AY, Canales FL, Furnas HJ. Why women request labiaplasty. Plast Reconstr Surg. 2017;139:856–63.
12. Moran C, Lee C. What's normal? Influencing women's perceptions of normal genitalia: an experiment involving exposure to modified and non modified images. BJOG. 2014;121:761–6.
13. Veale D, Eshkevari E, Ellison N, et al. Psychological characteristics and motivation of women seeking labiaplasty. Psychol Med. 2014;44:555–6.
14. Triana L, Robledo AM. Aesthetic surgery of female external genitalia. Aesthet Surg J. 2015;35(2):165–77.
15. Hamori CA, Banwell PE, Alinsod R. Female cosmetic genital surgery. Concept, classification and techniques. Spanish edition. Venezuela: AMOLCA, Actualidades Médicas CA; 2019.
16. Clerico C, Lari A, Mojallal A, Boucher F. Anatomy and aesthetics of labia minora: the ideal vulva? Aesthet Plast Surg. 2017;41(3):714–9.
17. Triana L. Commentary on Anatomy and aesthetics of the labia minora; the ideal vulva? Aesthet Plast Surg. 2017;41(4):993–4.
18. Ouar N, Gillier D, Moris V, Revol M, Francois C, Cristofaris S. Postoperative complications of labia minora reduction. Comparative study between wedge and edge resection. Ann Chir Plast Esthet. 2017;62(3):219, 223.
19. Sharp G, Tiggermann M, Mattiske J. Reply: Psychological outcomes of labiaplasty: a prospective study. Plast Reconstr Surg. 2017;140(3):507e–8e.
20. Martincik J, Malinovsky L. Surgical treatment of the hypertrophy of the labia minora. Cesk Gynekol. 1971;36:216–7. (article in Czech)
21. Radman HM. Hypertrophy of labia minora. Obstet Gynecol. 1976;48(1 Suppl):78s–9s.
22. Honoré LH, O'Hara KE. Benign enlargement of labia minora: report of two cases. Eur J Obstet Gynecol Reprod Biol. 1978;8(2):61–4.
23. Hodgkinson DJ, Hait G. Aesthetic vaginal labioplasty. Plast Reconstr Surg. 1984;74:314–416.
24. Alter GJ. A new technique for aesthetic labia minora reduction. Ann Plast Surg. 1998;40:287–90.
25. Motakef S, Rodriguez-Feliz J, Chung MT, Ingargiola MJ, Wong VW, Patel A. Vaginal labiaplasty: a systematic review, simplified classification system, and standardized practice guidelines. Plast Reconstr Surg. 2014;134:125–6.
26. Motakef S, Rodriguez-Feliz J, Chung MT, Ingargiola MJ, Wong VW, Patel A. Vaginal labiaplasty: current practices and a simplified classification system for labial protusion. Plast Reconstr Surg. 2015;135:774–85.
27. Furnas HJ. Trim labiaplasty. Plast Reconstr Surg Glob Open. 2017;5(5):e1349–54.
28. Chavis WM, LaFeria JJ, Niccolini R. Plastic repair of elongated, hypertrophic labia minora. A case report. J Reprod Med. 1989;34:373–5.
29. Felicio Y. Labial surgery. Aesthet Surg J. 2007;27:223–8.
30. Maas SM, Hage JJ. Functional and aesthetic labia minora reduction. Plast Reconstr Surg. 2000;105:1453–6.
31. Laufer MRG, Galvin WJ. Labia hypertrophy: a new surgical approach. Adolesc Pediatr Gynecol. 1995;8:3941.
32. Giraldo F, Gonzalez C, Haro F. Central wedge nymphectomy with 90-degree Z-plasty for aesthetic reduction of the labia minora. Plast Reconstr Surg. 2004;113:1820–5.
33. Rouzier RM, Louis-Sylvestre C, Paniel BJ, Haddad B. Hypertrophy of labia minora: experience with 163 reductions. Am J Obstet Gynecol. 2000;182:35–40.

34. Kelishadi SS, Elston J, Ran A, Tutela JP, Mizuguchi NN. Posterior wedge resection: a more aesthetic labiaplasty. Aesthet Surg J. 2013;33:847–53.
35. Munhoz AM, Filassi JR, Ricci MD, et al. Aesthetic labia minora reduction with inferior wedge resection and superior pedicle flap reconstruction. Plast Reconstr Surg. 2006;118:1237–47.
36. Choi H, Kim K. A new method for aesthetic reduction to the labia minora (the deepithelialized reduction labiaplasty). Plast Reconstr Surg. 2000;105:423–4.
37. Ostrzenski A. Fenestration labioreduction of the labium minus: a new surgical intervention concept. ISRN Obstet Gynecol. 2014;2014:671068.
38. Pardo J, Sola V, Ricci P, Guillof E. Laser labioplasty of labia minora. Int Gynaecol Obstet. 2006;93:38–43.
39. Smarrito S. Lambda laser nymphoplasty: retrospective study of 231 cases. Plast Reconstr Surg. 2014;133:231e–2e.
40. Gonzalez-Isaza P, Lotti T, Franca K, et al. Carbon dioxide with a new pulse profile and shape: a perfect tool to perform labiaplasty for functional and cosmetic purpose. Open Access Maced J Med Sci. 2018;6(1):25–7.
41. Ellsworth WA, Rizvi M, Lypka M, Gaon M, Smith B, Cohen B, Dinh T. Techniques for labia minora reduction: an algorithmic approach. Aesthet Plast Surg. 2010;34(1):105–10.
42. Veale D, Eshkevari E, Ellison N, et al. Validation of genital appearance satisfaction scale and the cosmetic procedure seeking scale women seeking labiaplasty. J Psychosom Obstet Gynaecol. 2013;34(1):46–52.
43. Veale D, Eshkevari E, Ellison N, et al. A comparison of risk factors for women seeking labiaplasty compared to those not seeking labiaplasty. Body Image. 2014;11:57–62.
44. Veale D, Naismith I, Eshkevari E, et al. Psychosexual outcome after labiaplasty: a prospective case-comparison study. Int Urogynecol J. 2014;25:831–9.
45. Mirzabeig MN, Moore JH Jr, Mericli AF, et al. Current trends in vaginal labioplasty: a survey of plastic surgeons. Ann Plast Surg. 2012;68:125–30.
46. Miklos JR, Moore RD. Postoperative cosmetic expectations for patients considering labiaplasty surgery: our experience with 550 patients. Surg Technol Int. 2011;21:170–4.
47. Alinsod R. Awake in-office Barbie labiaplasty, awake in-office labia majora plasty, awake in-office vaginoplasty, awake in-office labial revision, sutureless band reléase, awake in-office mesh excision, labia majora Pellevé. Presented at the Congress on Aesthetic vaginal Surgery. Tucson, AZ, Nov 2011.
48. Georgiou CA, Benatar M, Dumas P, et al. A cadaveric study of the arterial blood supply of the labia minora. Plast Reconstr Surg. 2015;136:167–78.
49. Lista F, Mistry BD, Singh Y, et al. The safety of aesthetic labiaplasty: a plastic surgery experience. Aesthet Surg J. 2015;35:689–95.

Chapter 6
Indications/Contraindications for Labiaplasty

Gustavo Adolfo Parra Solano

Introduction

As this book has written in many paragraphs, labiaplasty is a procedure that is increasing every day, "aesthetic procedures" are performed in the female external genitalia. But why is this increase in procedures? There may be several causes such as:

- Previously the trimming of pubic hair was not a custom, so the exposure of the vulvar anatomy was not evident; also patients did not explore their genitals frequently, probably associated with modesty and impositions given by society. With the passage of time fashions and customs change, so the trimming of genital hair began to become popular and later an habitual practice, the greater knowledge of anatomy of the genitals, plus all the advances in women's rights (which has led women to have a larger space in society, with increased confidence and changes in their preferences and needs).
- Now the expose of the vulvar appearance (given by the absence of hair), coupled with more information on the network (pornography, pictures of vulvas, etc.). It makes it easier for the patient to compare her genitalia with external imaging. In this way determining what she can consider as "normality or abnormality" [1].

Now I would like to clarify two terms that I used earlier which are "aesthetic procedures" and "normality or abnormality."

1. Aesthetic procedures: In the case of vulvo-vaginal surgery, the term aesthetic should not be used alone; the goal of surgery is to improve the functionality

G. A. P. Solano (✉)
Uroginecologia y Cirugia de Piso Pelvico, Hospital Universitario, SES Hospital de Caldas, Caldas, Colombia
e-mail: gustavo.parra@profamilia.org.co

© The Author(s), under exclusive license to Springer Nature Switzerland AG 2023
P. Gonzalez-Isaza, R. Sánchez-Borrego (eds.), *Topographic Labiaplasty*,
https://doi.org/10.1007/978-3-031-15048-7_6

associated with aesthetics; only in this way we will get the best results with our patients. The poor knowledge of anatomy and function from different structures will lead to complications such as mutilation, loss of function, pain, etc. Therefore, the goal with the knowledge acquired through books like this is to begin to perform surgeries aiming to preservation of "aesthetics-function."

2. Normality or abnormality: This is a very important term to clarify and that there are no normal or abnormal vulvas, all configurations of the vulva are different, and there are multiple shapes and sizes, for both labia minora majora, clitoral hood, and perineum. And depending on the characteristics, culture, and desire of the patient, you can be satisfied or not with the vulvar configuration.

With this brief introduction I want to give you some clear ideas that can guide which patient is the most suitable to undergo a surgical procedure (labiaplasty).

I do not want to point out a list of indications and contraindications; I want through this text to provide tools that help us choose the right indication for a labiaplasty.

Now going back to the beginning of this chapter, we talk about the increasing demand for vaginal cosmetic surgery. This increase in the number of procedures leads to practitioners without proper training to perform them. With the obvious consequences of "doing something without knowing how to do it," then I return to the concept of performing "cosmetic-functional" procedures; in order to perform a successful labiaplasty, the first thing we must know is the anatomy of the area; this includes (a) knowing the vulvar nerve supply; (b) knowing that there are four vascular branches of the vulva, called artery C, P1, P2, and A and what is the distribution of these in the labia minora [2]; and (c) knowing what different anatomical variations occur in the vulva. Second, to know the different techniques used in labiaplasty. Third, to know the material and instruments to use, which are the best sutures, which type to use or which is better (braided vs. monofilament), use of running and no running suture, the degree of tension of suture knots, tissue management, instruments suitable for use, etc. Fourth, have a training provided by experienced personnel, only this level of training can provide us with "pills" of knowledge that will make our procedure successful. Fifth, to know what are the complications, recovery time, post labiaplasty symptoms, post-surgical recommendations, etc. That will ultimately complement our comprehensive management of the patient.

In this case, we should apply the principles of medical ethics, called beneficence and non-maleficence, which are the principle of beneficence is that where the doctor who performs the procedure is familiar with it, knows the different techniques, and recognizes the anatomy of the area to be intervened. The principle of non-maleficence is one where we should not harm the patient; there are studies that show that cutting the labia minora does not affect the sensitivity of the area. Applying these two principles would give us a first indication to be able to intervene a patient. The obviation of the principle of beneficence by itself would affect the principle of non-maleficence; I explain "I know that cutting the labia minora does not affect the sensitivity, so I can do it. However, I do not know the techniques or the anatomy, by making this cut is likely to alter the functionality of the area, violating the two principles". Which specialist would be more qualified to perform this surgery; I would think that the one who is more familiar with pelvic surgery, this person would be more comfortable, more familiar with the anatomy. This person could be a gynecologist, a urologist, or a plastic surgeon with knowledge of anatomy and pelvic surgery [3, 4]. In case of untrained personnel without knowledge, I consider that is definitely a contraindication for labiaplasty. In the other hand body dysmorphic syndrome creates significant distress in the person and can alter their social, work, academic, or other functional performance. They may develop repetitive behaviors, such as looking in the mirror, comparing the disliked area with other people, etc.; in response to concerns about their appearance, it can be considered a relative contraindication for labiaplasty.

As mentioned in the previous paragraph, the patient may have an exaggerated concern for some non-obvious or slightly obvious defect. In case the patient has an anatomical variant susceptible to be taken to an aesthetic-functional correction, and we have a high suspicion of a body dysmorphic syndrome, we should initiate a multidisciplinary management before surgery (psychiatry and psychology), often after controlling the underlying disease the patient desists from surgery because she does not find her appearance as "unpleasant" as she thought before being treated.

Before going any further, I would like to bring up the definition of health, given by the World Health Organization (WHO). "*Health is a state of complete physical, mental and social well-being and not merely the absence of disease or infirmity.*" The quotation comes from the preamble of the constitution of the World Health Organization, which was adopted by the International Health Conference, held in New York from 19 June to 22 July 1946, signed on 22 July 1946 by the representatives of 61 states (official records of the World Health Organization, No. 2, p. 100), and entered into force on 7 April 1948. The definition has not been changed since 1948 [5].

I bring this definition to you because it is very likely that the patient's complaint is underestimated, with the excuse that the configuration of her genitalia does not put her health at risk or affect her health, and that the attempt to provide a solution to her discomfort is omitted.

This would be another indication to perform a labiaplasty; it would be the patient's desire for the procedure because of a complaint that affects her health and well-being.

In 2013, the Canadian Society of Obstetrics and Gynecology published a statement policy, where they did not recommend labiaplasty to patients. Within the article they provide some indications for vulvar or vaginal interventions, such as pelvic organ prolapse, postpartum perineal scarring, congenital malformations, or tumors. In case of "significant anatomical variations," reconstruction may be medically recommended [6].

But what is a significant anatomical variation, I think it is important to consider the views of each person; it is possible that a patient with a hypertrophy III-C-S (Gonzalez classification), perceive that their anatomy is not bothersome, is comfortable with their appearance and do not perceive any discomfort. However, another patient with an II-B-A hypertrophy is totally dissatisfied with her appearance, perceives discomfort, and/or affects her sexuality. Therefore, I consider that the term "significant anatomical variation" does not apply in the specific case of labia-plasty because of what I explained above. An indication would be then the desire of the patient to have an aesthetic-functional procedure, in the presence of labia minora hypertrophy.

From this indication we can deduce a contraindication. The patient must always desire and request the procedure, for the reasons that she considers that this ana-tomical variant affects her quality of life. But there are cases in which the procedure is requested by the patient's partner, since he is the one who considers that his part-ner does not have "normal" genitals. It is also necessary to investigate and suspect cases of sexual exploitation.

A contraindication would be the patient's unwillingness or coercion to undergo the procedure.

Now evaluating the reasons why the patient undergoes a labiaplasty, usually in the websites of surgeons one of the most exposed reasons is "for physical discom-fort associated with hypertrophy," however in a study [7], the reasons given in online communities (forums) by women were evaluated and compared with the reasons given on the websites of surgeons. The most frequent reason given by women in the forums was discomfort or emotional discomfort (71%), with a feeling of "mon-strous" appearance or aversion to their appearance, social embarrassment, fear, or during sexual intercourse there is fear of the reaction of the partner to the configura-tion of their genitals. This is followed by a search for improvement in functional discomfort, such as discomfort with wearing tight clothing, pain with intercourse, discomfort, or pain when riding a bicycle or dancing. A third reason is the postop-erative emotional improvement, feeling of normality, more attractive appearance, and improved sensations during sexual intercourse. Finally, and with a lower fre-quency (7.5%) was the functional improvement, seeking to improve hygiene and decrease friction with clothing.

Once compared with what was exposed on the websites of surgeons was found, the websites of surgeons showed 98% of the reasons for consultation of women was the emotional discomfort, however compared with what was reported in the forums was found to be 71%; also in the item functional discomfort websites reported an incidence of 90% vs. 52.5%, these with statistically significant differences, proba-bly indicating that what is published on the websites is not really the main com-plaints of patients.

During a gynecological consultation, it is not ethical to induce the patient to perform an aesthetic-functional procedure; we can only provide information if the patient requests it. Remember that vulvas are not normal or abnormal; they are all different and depending on the patient's perspective she may consider her labia to be "attractive" or on the contrary she may be dissatisfied with their configuration.

In some cultures, it is considered that long labia minora are sexually attractive, as is the case in some South African cultures. Where in early stages of life of women through techniques such as digital manipulation or use of weight on the labia minora manage to elongate these, preparing the woman before sexual initiation, with the concept that this labia minora configuration will improve sexual pleasure.

In another study, which sought to evaluate the size of the labia minora and the patient's perception of them, they took 244 measurements and applied a brief survey if they considered their labia to be normal or abnormal. They found that 54% of the patients had labia that protruded beyond the labia majora (visible). They also classified the labia according to their size. It is noteworthy that in patients who had labia larger than 25 mm, 66% considered their labia to be normal, the same occurred in those who had labia between 21 and 25 mm, where 75% of them considered their appearance to be normal [8].

It is a contraindication to induce the patient to undergo an aesthetic-functional procedure without her having requested it.

With respect to age, in Colombia according to the law, Law 1799 of 2016 of July 25 reads

- **ARTICLE 1. OBJECT.** The purpose of this law is to prohibit medical and cosmetic surgical procedures for underage patients and establish the penalty regime for those who violate this prohibition.
- **ARTICLE 2. DEFINITION.** For all the effects of the present law, aesthetic medical and surgical procedures shall be understood as any medical or surgical procedure of correction of alterations of the aesthetic norm with the purpose of obtaining a greater facial and corporal harmony, as well as medical treatments of beautification and rejuvenation.
- **ARTICLE 3. PROHIBITION.** The performance of aesthetic medical and surgical procedures on patients under 18 years of age is prohibited. Parental consent does not constitute a valid exception to this prohibition.
- **ARTICLE 4. EXCEPTIONS.** The above prohibition does not apply to nose and ear surgeries, reconstructive and/or iatrogenic surgeries of other surgeries, superficial chemical and mechanical peelings, and laser hair removal. Nor does it apply to surgeries motivated by physical or psychological pathologies duly accredited by the respective health professionals.

In cases of surgeries motivated by physical or psychological pathologies, the surgeon must request a special permit from the territorial health entity to perform the procedure [9].

However, the constitutional court ruled on this:

FIRST DEGREE -THE CONDITIONED EXEQUIBILITY, on the charges analyzed, of Article 3 of Law 1799 of 2016, on the understanding that the prohibition provided therein does not apply to adolescents over 14 years of age who have the evolutionary capacity, to participate with those who have parental authority in the decision about the risks assumed with this type of procedure and in compliance with informed and qualified consent. [10]

Analyzing the rules set out above, the law passed in 2016 allowed minors to undergo an aesthetic procedure, in case of reconstructive surgeries or previous iatrogenic procedures. With the pronouncement of the court, it was allowed that those over 14 years old can make the decision to undergo an aesthetic surgery, as long as they have the consent of their parents.

Now this is a rule of compliance in Colombia; each country has its own laws that allow or prohibit cosmetic procedures in minors; it is necessary to know the laws of our countries before taking a patient to a procedure.

Now I would like to clarify a couple of points:

- First, it has been emphasized that labiaplasty is an aesthetic-functional procedure, with which we seek to improve the health of the patient (remember the WHO definition of health) [5]. Therefore, we are not performing an aesthetic procedure as the only objective. In a study by Miklos and Moore, they found that the vast majority of patients who underwent labiaplasty did not have aesthetic improvement as the main reason, the vast majority did it looking to have a functional improvement, and almost never had coercion by another person [11].

- Second, while it is possible that the laws of our country allow surgery on minors, to what extent is it ethical to take the patient to a procedure in adolescence? Let us remember that the onset of adolescence is accompanied by an increase in circulating sex hormones, with maturation of the genitals and changes in their initial configuration. Many times, sexual life begins in these stages of life, which may favor the increase in size of the labia minora. There may be "irritative" processes, such as infections, heavy menstruation, use of genitalia piercings that affect both the color and the labial configuration, etc. If we perform a labiaplasty, it is likely that these changes mentioned above influence in a new growth of the labia minora, not reaching the primary objective of the intervention. With this I want to invite you to study each case in particular, modify the conditions that we suspect may affect the future procedure, avoid operating patients who have a genital development in process, and in case of defining to take the patient to a procedure explain clearly that by age, pregnancy, the onset of sexual intercourse genitalia may undergo changes again.

As a recommendation, avoid operating patients in their adolescence; in case you need to do it, you must provide all the necessary information and explain to the patient and her parents that may require a new procedure in adulthood or late adolescence.

Now let's remember that labiaplasty is a procedure that is under increasing demand, so it is likely that untrained people perform it, either because the patient requests it in a private consultation or is performed through health systems, As a result of this intervention performed by unskilled personnel, complications arise, known as "botched labiaplasty," as examples of this we can have amputation of labia minora, disinsertion of clitoral frenulum, lack of asymmetry by not intervening in the compartment I (clitoral hood), pain, etc. In this case the patient should be operated by someone with knowledge and experience in anatomy and female genital reconstruction, seeking to restore the anatomy and functionality of the area.

A clear indication for revision labiaplasty (we will call the re-intervention of a previous procedure) is that we will perform on previous failed procedures.

Knowing limits is important; it is likely that we have a training in labiaplasty, but we do not have the necessary experience. Or the patient has a very complex case that requires surgical techniques with which we are not familiar (fat grafting techniques, flap rotation, etc.). In this case recognizing our limits and being prudent is the best surgical decision we can make, seek support from our teachers and colleagues with more experience, or perform a multidisciplinary management will provide us with better results in our patients.

The procedure performed is as important as the postoperative control, within the control we can solve problems such as suture dehiscence, hematomas, infection, etc. We cannot ignore this in any way, so if the patient cannot follow up the postoperative period adequately, it is better not to perform the procedure.

Then a contraindication for labiaplasty is the impossibility of performing postoperative follow up to the patient.

To conclude this chapter and as I expressed at the beginning of this is not possible to provide you with a list of indications and contraindications, labiaplasty is a relatively new procedure, which is booming, but is discredited by many media and communities, as well as accepted by others. The correct decision-making, respect for the patient's wishes, responsibility in performing the surgery, acceptable aesthetic-functional results, and ethics will achieve greater acceptance in the community and medical associations of aesthetic-functional gynecologic surgery.

References

1. Mowat H, McDonald K, Dobson AS, Fisher J, Kirkman M, Mowat, et al. The contribution of online content to the promotion and normalisation of female genital cosmetic surgery: a systematic review of the literature. BMC Womens Health. 2015;15:110.
2. Goodman MP. Female genital cosmetic and plastic surgery: a review. J Sex Med. 2011;8:1813–25.
3. Pauls RN, Rogers RG, Rardin CR. Should gynecologists provide cosmetic labiaplasty procedures? Am J Obstet Gynecol. 2014;211(3):218.e1.
4. Church CB, Yurteri-Kaplan L, Alinsod R. Female genital cosmetic surgery: a review of techniques and outcomes. Int Urogynecol J. 2013; https://doi.org/10.1007/s00192-013-2117-8.
5. https://www.who.int/es.
6. Female genital cosmetic surgery. SOGC POLICY STATEMENT, No. 300; 2013.
7. Zwier S. "What motivates her": motivations for considering labial reduction surgery as recounted on women's online communities and surgeons' websites. Sex Med. 2014;2:16–23.
8. Lykkebo AW, Drue HC, Lam JUH, Guldberg R. The size of labia minora and perception of genital appearance: a cross-sectional study. J Low Genit Tract Dis. 2017;21(3)
9. http://www.secretariasenado.gov.co/senado/basedoc/ley_1799_2016.html.
10. https://www.corteconstitucional.gov.co/comunicados/No.%2022%20comunicado%2026%20de%20abril%20de%202017.pdf.
11. Miklos JR, Moore RD. Labiaplasty of the labia minora: patients' indications for pursuing surgery. J Sex Med. 2008;5:1492–5.

Chapter 7
Anesthetic Considerations for Labiaplasty

Othman Sulaiman

Introduction

Information on anesthetic considerations for labiaplasty is scarce, as the popularity of this surgical technique was not as widespread as it is today. It is not only considered a purely aesthetic procedure; it is also performed for functional reasons [1]. According to the NCEPOD classification of the procedure, labiaplasty is considered a scheduled elective procedure [2].

In a study involving 451 patients undergoing labiaplasty, the average age was 32.6 years (between 14 and 68 years) [3], but the majority of patients are between 19 and 50 years of age [4, 5]. We have a defined age group.

These are patients who undergo the procedure for multiple reasons such as external appearance related (aesthetic), functional not related to the sexual intercourse, or functional related to the sexual intercourse [3].

Pre-anesthetic Assessment

It will be performed according to the clinical practice manual on patient preparation for surgery of the Colombian Society of Anesthesiology [6].

The assessment should be aimed at determining the peculiarities of this age group. The surgical risk of labiaplasty is low risk (cardiovascular death and cardiac arrest at 30 days) less than 1%, according to Glance et al. [7]. It must be considered that in Colombia the legislation prohibits the performance of aesthetic surgeries to minors under 18 years of age with the exception of surgeries motivated by physical or psychological pathologies [8].

O. Sulaiman (✉)
Anesthesia Department, Liga Contra el Cáncer, Pereira, Risaralda, Colombia

© The Author(s), under exclusive license to Springer Nature Switzerland AG 2023
P. Gonzalez-Isaza, R. Sánchez-Borrego (eds.), *Topographic Labiaplasty*,
https://doi.org/10.1007/978-3-031-15048-7_7

The assessment should include at least the data on the type of procedure scheduled, the medical history, and the nutritional, respiratory and cardiovascular status. In general, they are patients with few or no pathological history; the main comorbidities described are anxiety, depression, and hypothyroidism [3]. Arterial hypertension and diabetes are less frequent.

The physical examination should include weight, height, and body mass index. It should also include vital signs, cardiorespiratory examination, and airway assessment.

Preclinical tests should be performed according to the findings of the clinical history and should not be rutinary in all patients. Inside our clinical practice, often patients do not require any blood tests.

The information given about the risks associated with the anesthetic act must be very clear, in simple language and that the patient and the family member fully understand; then obtain a signed informed consent [9].

It is of great importance to note the patient's anesthetic preferences in the clinical history. Since local, local sedation, regional spinal, or general anesthetic techniques have been described [5], the patient may be more attracted to a particular technique. This decision should be guided by the anesthesiologist who will recommend an alternative that suits the patient's special wishes and requirements.

Presurgical

Strict use will be made of the checklist recommended by the World Health Organization. Safety in surgery is essential. Adverse events in surgery are a major problem globally. Many are preventable. The WHO surgical safety checklist has been shown to reduce surgical complications and improve communication and teamwork in the operating room [10].

Three points are important to reduce intraoperative and postoperative complications: use of prophylactic antibiotics, avoidance of hypothermia, and assessment of the risk of venous thromboembolism (VTE).

For gynecological procedures and knowing the type of most common germs found inside the surgical area (gram-negative enteric bacilli, anaerobes, group B streptococcus, and enterococci), the use of cephalosporins (cefazolin, cefoxitin, cefotetan, or cefuroxime) or ampicillin-sulbactam is recommended. For patients with allergies, an alternative regimen with clindamycin + (ciprofloxacin or levofloxacin or gentamicin or aztreonam) is recommended [6].

Hypothermia triggers multiple complications. It is defined as a decrease in body temperature below 36 °C. Patients suffering from hypothermia may present decreased oxygen delivery to tissues, risk of arrhythmias, tendency to coagulopathies, worsening of electrolyte imbalance, oliguria, postoperative shivering, increased risk of surgical wound infection, and delayed healing [11]. For this reason, strategies should be implemented to reduce the risk of hypothermia (Table 7.1).

Table 7.1 Prevention of hypothermia in the preoperative and transoperative period

Intervention	Timing
Operating theater preheating	Presurgical
Preheating of patient with thermal blanket 1 h before the procedure	Presurgical
Heating of intravenous fluids in contact with the patient (local anesthetics, antiseptics, intravenous fluids)	Intra-surgical
Use of low flows in the anesthesia and humidifier circuits	Intra-surgical
Use of thermal blankets	Intra-surgical
Covering of exposed body parts	Intra-surgical

Table 7.2 Preoperative estimation of venous thromboembolism risk

Factor de riesgo	Puntos
Age > 60 years	1
Body mass index > 40 kg/m^2	1
Male gender	2
Septic shock	3
Personal history of VTE	3
Familiar history of VTE	4
Cancer	5

Minimal risk, 0 points; low risk, 1–2 points; moderate risk, 3–5 points; high risk, (≥6 points) (modified from [6])

Patients with VTE have unacceptable short-term mortality and long-term morbidity, and it is responsible for the death of more than 100,000 people annually in the United States [12].

VTE risk staging should be performed preoperatively. There are several predictive models for staging this condition, but the most widely used at present is that of Pannucci et al. [13], which is easy and agile to use, is concrete, and has few variables to evaluate (Table 7.2).

In a systematic review of the literature on methods to avoid VTE in bariatric surgery patients [14], and which can be extended to other surgical procedures such as labiaplasty, several alternatives are listed such as early ambulation, use of elastic compression stockings or intermittent pneumatic compression stockings, pharmacological prophylaxis with anticoagulants, and in other cases the use of vena cava filters.

In the context of labiaplasty, non-pharmacological and pharmacological methods are the most commonly used, all depending on the specific context of each patient. The use of vena cava filters is left to patients at high risk of VTE or pulmonary embolism who cannot be anticoagulated. Per se, these patients are not suitable for labiaplasty.

There are other associated complications, which are relatively frequent and are summarized in Table 7.3 [15].

Table 7.3 Summary of the most frequent complications in anesthesia[a]

Category	Troubleshooting	Potential clinical outcomes
Airway	Difficult intubation	Dental trauma Soft tissues trauma Hypoxia
	No intubation, no oxygenation	Hypoxia Airway trauma Surgery cancellation Death
Ventilatory	Airway high pressure	Lung barotrauma Pneumothorax
	Endobronchial intubation Bronchial aspiration	Hypoxia Pneumonitis Prolonged ventilation
Cardiovascular	Hypotension	Myocardial ischemia Cardiac arrest Brain injury
	Hypertension	Bleeding Stroke Aneurism rupture
Central and peripheral nervous system	Intraneural injection	Peripheral nerve lesion Weakness Pain
	Dural punction Failure to activate vaporizer	Post-puncture headache Intraoperative awakening Psychological trauma
Medicamentos	Allergies Idiosyncratic reaction Failures of administration Endovenous line failure	Anaphylaxis Malignant hyperthermia Miscellaneous effects: hypertension, neuromuscular block Intraoperative awakening Failure of medication effects Compartment syndrome Tissue necrosis

[a] Modified from Merry [15]

Brief Description of the Most Commonly Used Anesthetic Techniques

Literature reviews describe techniques with local anesthesia under sedation and general anesthesia, the latter mainly in patients undergoing additional surgical procedures. The most commonly described local anesthetics are 1% lidocaine with epinephrine 1:200,000; 0.5% lidocaine with epinephrine 1:200,000; and 0.25% bupivacaine with epinephrine 1:200,000 or 1:50,000 [5].

In our clinical practice, and from our experience, we are more inclined to use general anesthesia and occasionally the use of regional spinal anesthesia. Subjectively, patients present more postoperative satisfaction than with local anesthetic techniques, without excluding them.

- Regional spinal anesthesia: Strict asepsis and antisepsis and spinal needle selection. Verification of intrathecal needle location and administration of local anesthetic (bupivacaine heavy 0.5%), adjuvants such as opioids can be administered. Verification of sensory blockade.
- Balanced general anesthesia: After preoxygenation of the patient, anesthetic induction will be performed. The choice of the type of airway device (supraglottic or infraglottic) will be at the doctor's discretion. We prefer the use of a laryngeal mask because it has many advantages: easy placement, does not require neuromuscular relaxants in most cases, avoids the neuroendocrine response of intubation, less trauma and postoperative pain, less incidence of cough or laryngospasm, and is cost-effective [16].

Medications:

- Propofol bolus 2–3 mg/kg
- Opioid: bolus fentanyl 2–3 μg/kg or remifentanil at 0.5–1 μg/kg
- Neuromuscular relaxant: succinylcholine 1–2 mg/kg, rocuronium 0.6–1.2 mg/kg or cisatracurium 0.1 mg/kg. The use of neuromuscular relaxant is preferred when infraglottic devices are used in airway management.

Maintenance of anesthesia will be done with sevoflurane at 0.8 MAC and remifentanil at 0.2–0.5 μg/kg/min.

Antiemetics and analgesics will be administered, if possible multimodal analgesia and avoiding the use of opioid agents.

Our patients are in the risk group for postoperative nausea and vomiting (Table 7.4). Therefore, it is imperative to take measures to prevent their occurrence.

The antiemetic regimen most commonly used by us is dexamethasone 4–8 mg in single dose and ondansetron 4–8 mg single dose, avoiding the use of long-acting opioids, and in selected patients it is possible to use total intravenous anesthesia substituting the inhaled agent with propofol in infusion [17].

During the procedure analgesia is of special importance. During the procedure we use multimodal analgesia (combination of agents that we have available

Table 7.4 Risk factors for postoperative nausea and vomiting

Category	Risk factors
Patient related	Female gender Previous history of nausea and vomits in postsurgical Nausea and vomits during car travels Age < 50 years
Anesthesia related	Prolonged anesthesia Pre- and postsurgical uses of opioids Use of volatile anesthetic agents Uses of neostigmine over 3 mg
Surgery related	Prolonged surgical procedures Type of surgery: neurosurgery, intra-abdominal surgery Laparoscopic surgery, gynecological surgery

Modified from Cao et al. [17]

maximizing analgesia and decreasing doses of individual drugs, which generates fewer adverse effects) [18]. The most commonly used combination in our patients is local anesthesia, nonsteroid analgesic, and acetaminophen or dipyrone, with excellent results. The use of opioids is very occasional; these are reserved for patients with low pain threshold or those who have undergone additional surgeries in the same anesthetic time.

In recovery rooms, measures will be taken to maintain well-being and comfort (oxygenation, normothermia, pain management).

Discharge, if no complications occur, with general recommendations. The most common analgesic regimen is a combination of acetaminophen and a nonsteroidal anti-inflammatory drug.

In conclusion, anesthesia for labiaplasty is very versatile, given the multiple ways of dealing with each particular case. Not neglecting the patient's preferences and having an empathic communication with the patient and the surgical team will make the success of the anesthetic procedure complete and satisfactory.

References

1. Miklos JR, Moore RD. Labiaplasty of the labia minora: patients' indications for pursuing surgery. J Sex Med. 2008;5(6):1492–5.
2. National Confidential Enquiry into Patient Outcome and Death [Internet]. http://www.ncepod.org.uk/.
3. Bucknor A, Chen AD, Egeler S, Bletsis P, Johnson AR, Myette K, Lin SJ, Hamori CA. Labiaplasty: indications and predictors of postoperative sequelae in 451 consecutive cases. Aesthet Surg J. 2018;38(6):644–53.
4. Cosmetic surgery national data bank statistics. Aesthet Surg J. 2018;38(Suppl_3):1–24.
5. Motakef S, Rodriguez-Feliz J, Chung MT, Ingargiola MJ, Wong VW, Patel A. Vaginal labiaplasty: current practices and a simplified classification system for labial protrusion. Plast Reconstr Surg. 2015;135(3):774–88.
6. Rincon-Valenzuela D, Escobar B. Evidence-based clinical practice manual: preparation of the patient for the surgical act and transfer to the operating room. Rev Colomb Anesthesiol. 2015;43(1):32–50.
7. Glance LG, Lustik SJ, Hannan EL, Osler TM, Mukamel DB, Qian F, Dick AW. The Surgical Mortality Probability Model: derivation and validation of a simple risk prediction rule for noncardiac surgery. Ann Surg. 2012;255(4):696–702.
8. Law 1799, which prohibits cosmetic medical and surgical procedures for minors and establishes other provisions. July 25, 2016. Republic of Colombia, National Government.
9. Ibarra P, Robledo B, Galindo M, Niño C, Rincón D. Minimum standards 2009 for the practice of anesthesiology in Colombia Safety Committee. Rev Colomb Anestesiol. 2009;37(3):235–53.
10. Woodman N, Walker I. World Health Organization surgical safety checklist. Patient Saf. 2016;2016:tutorial 325. www.wfshaq.org
11. Nath SS, Roy D, Ansari F, Pawar ST. Anaesthetic complications in plastic surgery. Indian J Plast Surg. 2013;46(2):445–52.
12. Centers for Disease Control and Prevention (CDC). Venous thromboembolism in adult hospitalizations - United States, 2007–2009. MMWR Morb Mortal Wkly Rep. 2012;61(22):401–4.
13. Pannucci CJ, Laird S, Dimick JB, Campbell DA, Henke PK. A validated risk model to predict 90-day VTE events in postsurgical patients. Chest. 2014;145(3):567–73.

14. Bartlett MA, Mauck KF, Daniels PR. Prevention of venous thromboembolism in patients undergoing bariatric surgery. Vasc Health Risk Manag. 2015;11:461–77.
15. Merry AF, Mitchell SJ. Complications of anaesthesia. Anaesthesia. 2018;73(Suppl 1):7–11.
16. Zaballos M, López S. Practical recommendations for the use of the laryngeal mask in outpatient surgery. Cir May Amb. 2008;13(1):4–26.
17. Cao X, White PF, Ma H. An update on the management of postoperative nausea and vomiting. J Anesth. 2017;31(4):617–26.
18. Nimmo SM, Foo ITH, Paterson HM. Enhanced recovery after surgery: pain management. J Surg Oncol. 2017;116(5):583–91.

Chapter 8
Surgical Instrumentation in Labiaplasty

Ana Maria Gutierrez

Surgical instrumentation is the art of mastering, creating, and manipulating all the instruments and supplies necessary to perform a surgical procedure.

It requires time, discipline, and concentration to obtain the best results before, during, and after surgery, having as a fundamental principle the safety of the patient and the whole surgical team.

Identifying the patient's needs provides on time, safe, and effective care with excellent results.

The main function of the surgical assistant is to guarantee reliable and safe sterilization processes and good management of the surgical technique, protocols, and the checklist established for the procedure, in addition to optimizing the requirements of supplies, elements, and instruments [1].

For labiaplasty we require cutting instruments including scalpel handle with 15 blade, standard 10 cm Steven's scissors, standard 10 cm Iris scissors, both scissors are designed to provide a firm grip while cutting with precision, and Mayo scissors or material scissors (Fig. 8.1).

Apprehension instrument including fine dissection Adson with and without claw, with its serrated and pointed end, allows to attract, approximate, and compress fine tissues.

Mayo Hegar needle holder, which is straight with a type of zipper to hold the needle, has concavities and grooves so that the needle does not move and allows the needle to pass through the tissues with precision.

Hemostatic instrumentation including curved mosquito forceps, which allows to compress small blood vessels and to hold suture ends for repairs (Fig. 8.1).

Among the supplies we use are the following:

Gauze, these are always counted at the beginning and at the end of surgery.

Swabs which we use to make tissue marking with the help of methylene blue.

A. M. Gutierrez (✉)
Surgical Assistancy Department, Calculaser Private Clinic, Pereira, Risaralda, Colombia

P. Gonzalez-Isaza, R. Sánchez-Borrego (eds.), *Topographic Labiaplasty*,
https://doi.org/10.1007/978-3-031-15048-7_8

Fig. 8.1 Surgical table, elements for labiaplasty

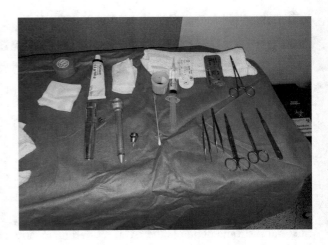

Flask or cuvette to deposit methylene blue.

Syringes of 10 and 20 mm.

27-gauge needle for tissue infiltration.

Stochette which is a tubular plastic roll that is used to dress the arm of the laser equipment and thus preserve its sterility for handling this biomedical equipment.

Saline solution 500 mL.

Compresses.

Gloves of different sizes.

Surgical clothing designed to separate the sterile area of the non-sterile decreasing the risk of infection can be made of polypropylene and/or woven fabric such as antifluid or cotton; both qualities must meet certain characteristics such as be fluid repellent, not be conductive of energy, light and easy to handle and a considerable size that sufficiently covers the surgical field, comfortable and hypoallergenic, and is not visible without perforations.

Sutures:

Vicryl 4-0 rapid: It is a colorless coated braided structure, composed of copolymer of polyglactin 910 (glycolide 90%, lactic 10%) of low molecular weight, with a 50% coating of polyglactin 370 (glycolide 35%, lactic 65%), and 50% of calcium stearate. It has a tensile strength retention profile of 50% in 5 days and 0% in 14 days, an absorption at 42 days. Its main uses include skin and mucosal closure, episiotomies, oral mucosa, conjunctiva, phimosis, and ligatures [2].

Monosyn 5-0: synthetic absorbable suture composed of glyconate (copolymer of glycolic acid (72%), epsilon, caprolactone (14%) and trimethylene carbonate (14%)), monofilament. It has 50% of the initial resistance after 14 days (useful resistance period) and 0% of the initial resistance (tensile strength) after 28 days.

Complete absorption of the mass (by hydrolysis) within 60–90 days.

It is used in thin tissues or potentially septic surgeries or in contact with urinary or digestive tract fluids; this suture has many advantages such as it gives security to the knotting, it has an excellent approach to the edges of the wound without altering its irrigation by the flexibility of its texture, and in addition this allows a smooth and atraumatic passage through the tissues.

Chromed Catgut 5-0: It is a natural absorbable suture, composed of purified connective tissue mainly collagen, derived from the serous layer of cattle (bovine) or the submucosal fibrous layer of the intestines of sheep (ovine); this type of suture is processed to provide greater resistance to absorption; its presentation comes in a solution that presents glycerol. Tensile retention profile of 21–28 days and an absorption time of 90 days, it has great resistance to knotting; when passing through the tissues due to its monofilament structure, it is absorbed by an enzymatic degradation.

Silk 2-0: It is of natural nonabsorbable origin made of fibroin which is a protein derived from the larva of the silkworm and is a black braided multifilament, for its great flexibility allows the passage through the tissues without causing greater damage and gives better handling and ease for knotting; in labiaplasty we use this type of sutures to make repairs of tissues.

The result of the labiaplasty is due to the updated knowledge, experience, and commitment of each member of the surgical team that makes it possible to perform the surgery, providing the patient safety inside the procedure, with high levels of quality, using appropriate scientific and technological criteria.

References

1. Fuller JR. Surgical instrumentation. Principles and practice. 3rd ed. Madrid: Panamericana; 1998.
2. Kudur M, Pai S, Sripathi H, Prabhu S. Sutures and suturing techniques in skin closure. Indian J Dermatol Venereol Leprol. 2009;75(4):425. https://doi.org/10.4103/0378-6323.53155.

Chapter 9
The Role of EBD Energy Sources in Performing Labiaplasty

Pablo Gonzalez-Isaza

Labiaplasty has been performed for more than four decades with traditional surgical technique scissors and scalpel; however the advancement of medical knowledge and technology of energy-based devices has motivated its use; my first experience was during a training course in the city of Santiago de los Caballeros, around the year 2007, when I was still a resident of gynecology and obstetrics second year in the military central hospital in Bogota, Colombia.

On this occasion I had the opportunity to perform labiaplasty on real patients, with a 980 nm diode laser equipment, with contact fiber; the procedure seemed to be easy and reproducible, with minimal bleeding and apparently an adequate recovery; unfortunately I never had a feedback about the postoperative evolution, neither aesthetic results. When I returned to Colombia and finished my training as a specialist, I returned to my hometown Pereira, where I found that a pulmonologist colleague had a similar equipment, which I rented and began to perform my first procedures; from the beginning it recalled my attention the important thermal damage and the edges with carbonization that generated the use of this technology, and therefore the postoperative results were not the best, from the point of view of pain, suture dehiscence, prolonged down time, and even worse the aesthetic results were not favorable (Fig. 9.1), given my curiosity I had the idea of using different sources of energy for performing a labiaplasty, such as mechanical energy (harmonic

Supplementary Information The online version contains supplementary material available at [https://doi.org/10.1007/978-3-031-15048-7_9].

P. Gonzalez-Isaza (✉)
Obstetrics and Gynecology Urogynecology Minimally Invasive Surgery Functional Cosmetic and Regenerative Gynecology, Hospital Universitario San Jorge/Liga contra el Cancer, Pereira, Madrid, Spain

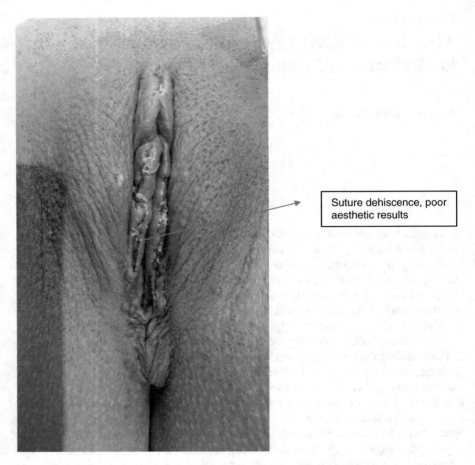

Suture dehiscence, poor aesthetic results

Fig. 9.1 Suture dehiscence related to excess of thermal effect of 980 Nm (diode laser)

scalpel), monopolar energy, high-frequency energy; I sent the surgical specimens to the pathology department asking the pathologist to examine under the microscope the lateral thermal damage generated by these different sources of energy; to my surprise I found that all these alternatives generated an important collateral thermal damage, which was clinically correlated with unfavorable outcomes, as well as poor aesthetic results (Table 9.1; Fig. 9.2).

Finally, towards the year 2011 during our I Latin American Symposium of Cosmetic Gynecology, I had the opportunity to learn about the best possible technology for performing this procedure, the CO_2 laser with multipulse emission system; we performed in vivo surgeries obtaining very satisfactory results, thanks to its versatility in terms of cutting and coagulation.

Table 9.1 Different energy sources with their respective collateral thermal damage in mm

Energy source	Thermal lateral damage pathology report (mm)
Monopolar ElectroCauterium	6
Radiofrequency (conization loops)	3
Harmonic scalpel	4
Diode laser	3
CO_2 laser	0.6–0.9 HP/SP/DP

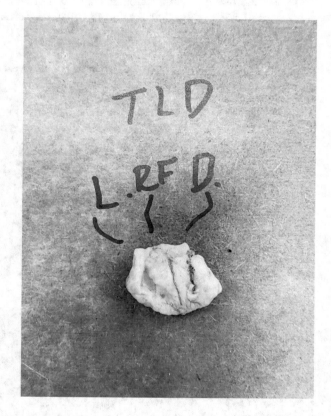

Fig. 9.2 Thermal effect on human vagina specimens from different energy sources, from left to right. L (pulsed CO_2 laser), RF (radio frequency), D (diode laser). Note the non-perceptible thermal effect of the pulsed CO_2 laser on the left, in the middle the RF with a carbonization effect, and undoubtedly greater tissue damage, with the diode laser on the right.

Subsequently in our published series, we demonstrated the versatility and safety of the Smart Xide 2 platform (Deka Laser Florence Italy), which allows the use of different pulse modes, according to the characteristics of the tissue, vascularization, and the degree of complexity of the cases of labia minora hypertrophy; in addition this tool provides greater precision at the time of cutting [1]; inside our laboratory we performed histological studies, comparing the different pulse modes, with its corresponding collateral thermal effect, thus concluding that the pulses with less thermal effect, such as HP, UP are the most suitable for performing a labiaplasty; however it should be noted that it requires a significant learning curve, to use this type of tools (Figs. 9.3, 9.4, 9.5, and 9.6).

From the point of view of postoperative results, we find, less postoperative pain, less analgesic requirement, and a short period of incapacity, the laser offers multiple advantages that justify its use for the benefit of patients in this type of surgical procedures (Fig. 9.7) [2].

Table 9.2 shows the complication rates in series of labiaplasty, showing a rate of dehiscence of 5.3%, related to a significant collateral thermal damage, by the use of diode laser (955 nm).

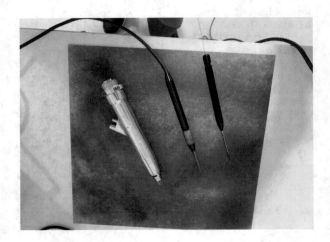

Fig. 9.3 Different energy sources, used from left to right. L (pulsed CO_2 laser), RF (radio frequency), D (diode laser)

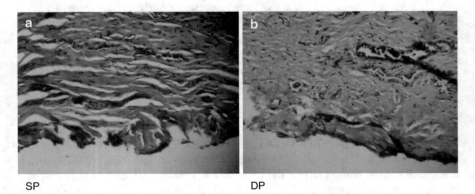

SP   DP

Fig. 9.4 Differences in thermal effect between two pulses (**a**) 0.5 mm (**b**) 0.8 mm

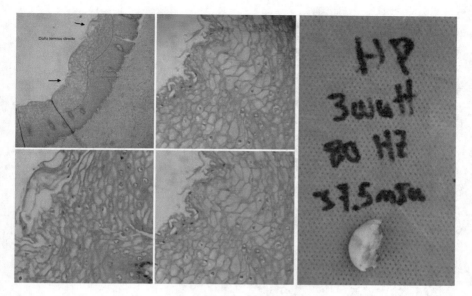

Fig. 9.5 Nearly no effect of the HP pulse on a fresh human vaginal specimen, hematoxylin-eosin staining

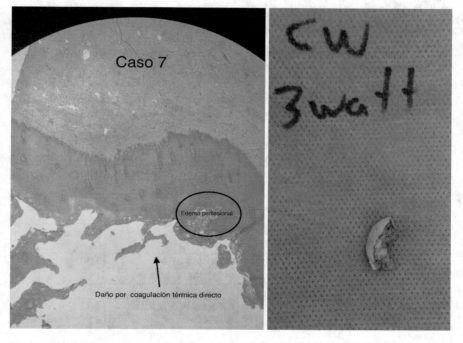

Fig. 9.6 Thermal effect of a continuous emission of pulsed CO_2 laser (CW) that generates carbonization in a specimen of fresh human vagina, hematoxylin-eosin staining

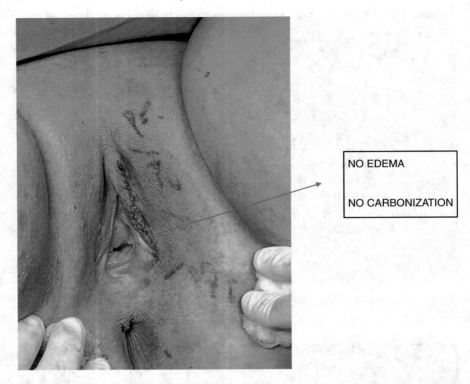

NO EDEMA

NO CARBONIZATION

Fig. 9.7 Immediate postoperative image of a linear labiaplasty with anatomical variant approach in the horizontal plane (bifurcation of the clitoral hood)

Table 9.2 Complication rates in series of labiaplasty, specifically Pardo and colleagues found a rate of dehiscence of 5.3%, related to a significant collateral thermal damage, by the use of diode laser (955 nm)

Author	# Pts	Follow up (months)	Technique	% Dehiscence
Hodgkinson/Hait 1984	3	60	Linear	0
Alter 1988	4	NA	V-wedge	0
Mass/Hage 2000	13	72	Linear	7.6
Choi/Kim 2000	6	NA	CHOI	0? Abandoned technique
Rouzier et al. 2000	163	30	Posterior wedge	7.0
Giraldo et al. 2004	15	30	V-ALTER	13.3
Pardo et al. 2006	55	2	Linear **Laser**	5.3
Munhoz et al. 2006	21	46	LINEAR POSTERIOR WEDGE	5.3 9.5
Alter 2008	**407**	NA	Vwedge + Clitoral Hood	2.9

References

1. González-Isaza P, Lotti T, França K, et al. Carbon dioxide with a new pulse profile and shape: a perfect tool to perform labiaplasty for functional and cosmetic purpose. Open Access Maced J Med Sci. 2018;6(1):25–7. https://doi.org/10.3889/oamjms.2018.043.
2. Adelman MR, Tsai LJ, Tangchitnob EP, Kahn BS. Laser technology and applications in gynaecology. J Obstet Gynaecol. 2013;33(3):225–31. https://doi.org/10.3109/0144361 5.2012.747495.

Chapter 10
Complications, How to Predict and Avoid Them

Pablo Gonzalez-Isaza

Labiaplasty is one of the most requested genital rejuvenation procedures today; the increase of labiaplasty goes in direct line with the increase of complications, in recent years has increased the number of revision or secondary labiaplasties [1] (Fig. 10.1). According to the American Association of Plastic and Cosmetic Surgeons, there was an increase in the number of labiaplasty procedures of 217% between 2012 and 2017 [2].

The number of procedures is estimated to increase by 15–20% each year.

The labia minora labiaplasty is the most common procedure and is part of more than 90% of surgeries at genital level; unfortunately we do not have epidemiological data for Latin American population [3]; recent literature has shown a trend in the

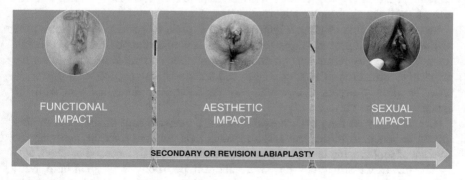

Fig. 10.1 Impact related to failed labiaplasty

P. Gonzalez-Isaza (✉)
Obstetrics and Gynecology Urogynecology Minimally Invasive Surgery Functional Cosmetic and Regenerative Gynecology, Hospital Universitario San Jorge/Liga contra el Cancer, Pereira, Madrid, Spain

variation of the reasons why a patient requests a labiaplasty [4]. Bucknor and collaborators in their series of 451 patients with a 7 years follow-up reported a rate of postoperative complications of 7.1% of which 3.8% were related to suture dehiscence with the central or wedge technique; the indication for revision labiaplasty in this group of patients was decided due to aesthetic discomfort and secondary sexual dysfunction [4].

Smarrito and collaborators in their article are emphatic in emphasizing that a poorly performed labiaplasty negatively impacts the aesthetics, functionality, and sexuality of patients [5].

In our experience, evaluating retrospectively, we have noticed that a possible complication can be avoided, even from the same initial consultation, in which the complaint, or the reason for consultation, should be properly evaluated. The main reasons for consultation of a woman with hypertrophy of the labia minora are as follows:

- Emotional
- Functional
- Behavioral
- Social
- Sexual

Once the complaint is evaluated, we proceed with an adequate identification of the patient's expectations; at this moment false expectations can be identified and if we apply appropriate questionnaires added to a good interrogation, it is possible to identify causes of body dysmorphic syndrome [6]; in the group of 55 patients that underwent labiaplasty by Veale and collaborators, they identified 10 that fulfilled criteria for body dysmorphic syndrome [7].

Additionally, it is of utmost importance to explain that it is possible to require additional surgical procedures or second look, as well as the possibility of presenting postsurgical asymmetries, which in our experience do not exceed 15%; for the physical examination, it is advisable to use a camera, colposcope, or a mirror, in order to allow the patient to adequately describe their dissatisfaction with the appearance of the vulva.

Continuing with the physical examination, a measurement of the labia minora should be made, in its vertical and horizontal axis, without traction, applying the concept of topographic labiaplasty measurement, previously exposed in Chap. 4.

The use of classifications for labia minora hypertrophy is of great help, but I believe that emphasis should be placed on the concept of topographic labiaplasty, the subject of this book, since it allows us not only to identify the components of labia minora hypertrophy but also to make a mental scheme and plan the best surgical technique that preserves the anatomy, sexuality, and functionality.

Once identified the components of labia minora hypertrophy, it is important to discuss with the patient their preferences, for example, there is a group of patients who prefer to preserve the edge of labia minora, which is why they could not perform a linear labiaplasty, but would have to perform different techniques such as central or wedges. On the other hand, if the patient does not want to preserve the edge of the labia because it is pigmented or has friction changes, then a technique that can resect the edge as trimming, linear, or lazy s should be selected.

In a labia minora hypertrophy scenario, there should always be room to discuss nonsurgical alternatives in patients who so desire. On the other hand, we should never induce a labiaplasty in a patient whose reason for consultation is different.

It is important to have photographic evidence of all cases before and after the procedure, in different views (cephalocaudal, lateral, and frontal) (Figs. 10.2 and 10.3).

For capturing these images, ideally use a professional camera (not mobile phones), always use the same type of lighting and settings in before and after photos, use a blue background, and most importantly that you have the authorization, by the patient for the images, in the informed consent (see informed consent model

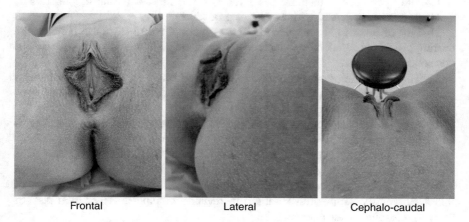

| Frontal | Lateral | Cephalo-caudal |

Fig. 10.2 Photos before frontal, lateral, cephalocaudal

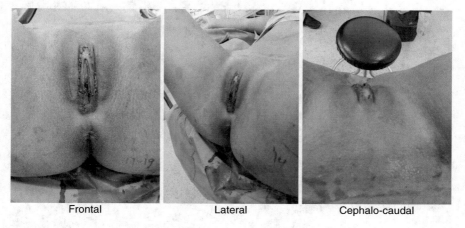

| Frontal | Lateral | Cephalo-caudal |

Fig. 10.3 Immediate postoperative photos

in the attachments section); this informed consent must have the following sections, so that the patient has the option to select which aspects authorizes.

- Authorization to take photos and videos to support the medical history
- Authorization to take photos and videos for academic and research purposes
- Authorization to take photos and videos for eventual publication and presentation in academic events

In our experience of more than 14 years, we have identified red flags (red alerts), which allow us to take actions and decisions that have an important impact on the possibility of complications.

Patients with a history of depression or anxiety (increased risk of body dysmorphic syndrome).

Couple dysfunction (in these cases most of the time, a sexual dysfunction is masked) that is not solved with a surgical procedure.

History of tobacco abuse, drug addiction, alcohol abuse (in these patients the healing process is deficient, and there is a higher rate of suture dehiscence and poor postsurgical results).

Patients requesting labiaplasty due to pressure from partners, peers, or parents (this group of patients is usually happy with the appearance of their vulva and does not require a surgical procedure).

Patients who request multiple procedures in the same surgical act related to genital aesthetics (higher risk of body dysmorphic syndrome).

Patients with repetitive questions about budget and costs of the procedure (this type of patients has a wrong perception of the cost-quality relationship).

Patients with a history of previous genital procedures, with the exception of failed labiaplasty, amputations, requiring revision labiaplasty (increased risk of body dysmorphic syndrome) (Fig. 10.4).

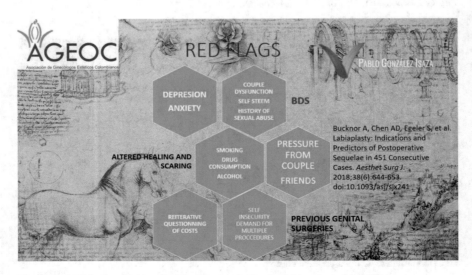

Fig. 10.4 Red flags to be identified in the consultation for labia minora hypertrophy

Currently, every good or service is valued more for the whole experience that was generated around it, than the outcome or final result, for example, if we go to dinner at a restaurant, the food was not to our liking, but the attention and all the service around the dinner were adequate; this remains in the memory of the consumer as an experience, and for this reason I dare to extrapolate to the labiaplasty.

Patient's First Access to the Labiaplasty Office

The labiaplasty is an intimate procedure, which generates embarrassment, shame, and discomfort; from the first call to request consultation, there must be a receptionist or secretary trained with the procedure, so adequate information is provided.

At the Time of Consultation

It should use a clear and friendly language that the patient can understand and use graphics or diagrams that can illustrate the condition; I reiterate the physical examination should be performed with a colposcope camera or mirror; the patient should be informed about the surgical plan, options the possibility of complications, asymmetries, poor results, etc., and at that time an informed consent must be provided (Table 10.1); in the same way as soon as possible schedule an appointment for preanesthetic assessment, in order to resolve doubts, discuss previous bad experiences, and decide the best anesthetic plan, with respect to the anesthesiologist, ideally should always be the same, as this allows standardize protocols, and so the experience is more reproducible.

Table 10.1 Labiaplasty consultation aspects

	CONSULTATION
ACCESS	Detailed
TRAINED ASSISTANT	Expectatives
PRECISE INFORMATION	Language
How did you find us?	Graphics/Photos
	Doubts

Peri-surgical Aspects

Ideally you should choose an accredited center, preferably located within a medical-hospital complex, as this can provide safety to patients; access should have the possibility of having a private area; the staff of the center should also be trained in this type of procedure; within the area of preoperative preparation, there should be no other patients from other specialties, neither male patients (Table 10.2).

Once the patient enters the operating room or procedures, all staff involved in the surgical procedure must be properly presented to the patient; I remember in my internship at the Santa Fe Foundation in Bogota between 2004 and 2005, I had the opportunity to enter as the first assistant to a procedure of dermo-lipectomy, with Professor Felipe Coifmann, great authority of Latin American plastic surgery (peace in his grave); in that opportunity Dr. Coifmann required that all staff be identified with full name and surname and additionally should inform the role in the surgery to be performed.

It is important to close the doors of the operating room and limit the entrance to personnel who are not related to the surgical procedure; it is not uncommon for personnel from other rooms to enter repeatedly to extract supplies or some type of elements, altering the privacy of the patient.

Table 10.2 Peri-surgical aspects

Peri-surgical aspects
Access to the center
Pre Anesthesia Appointment
Personnel

Operating Room

Prior to the anesthesia, it is important to perform a physical examination again and confirm with the surgical team as a checklist, the procedure and technique to be performed, in our experience has not been uncommon to find patients requesting additional procedures, what I call (bonus). It is important to clarify to the patient that any procedure that has not been previously discussed in the outpatient clinic, which is not consigned in the informed consent, ideally should not be performed, and that it is not the best time to make such decisions, not only because the patient could be under premedication protocol but also because we have more undesired outcomes when such conduct is adopted (Table 10.3).

Once the anesthesia is started, we proceed to evaluate again the clinical characteristics of the labia minora hypertrophy, and at that moment we proceed to perform our first marking following the guidelines of topographic labiaplasty.

Table 10.3 Operating room aspects

Operating theater
Non Planned procedures (No bonus)
Photos—Videos
Privacy
Markings
Doubts

Recovery

During the recovery process in order to have a more appropriate and pleasant recovery, there must be an adequate analgesic plan and local media, such as ice or cold compresses, we must be very careful with the hallway comments regarding the case, and finally there must be an adequate match with the postsurgical recommendations delivered in the consultation, with those handed to the patient inside the operating room (Table 10.4).

The recovery process also includes an adequate telephone follow-up, if possible the same night and the next day, must be supported with an adequate questionnaire with standardized questions that reflect the recovery process, that can identify possible complications in the early recovery period; it is very important to clarify to patients, that the final result may take up to 6 months (Table 10.5).

When a face-to-face follow-up is not possible because the patients are foreigners, a video call should be made with encrypted platforms, and the information should be recorded in the clinical history.

During these visits, inflammation, bleeding, hematomas, symmetry, and reaction to the suture material should be evaluated.

In summary, it is important to have an adequate doctor-patient relationship in which open communication is possible, treatment options can be discussed, and risk factors for body dysmorphic syndrome can be identified. If the reason for consultation coincides with the physical examination, and the indication is in accordance with the patient's expectations, the probability of having a negative outcome is extremely rare (Fig. 10.5).

Table 10.4 Recovery aspects

Post surgical
Coherence for after care recommendations
Pain management/ice
Privacy
Prudency with information

Table 10.5 Postsurgical follow-ups

1 Week	2 Weeks	4 Weeks	12 Weeks	6 Months	12 Months
Inflammation	Suture reaction	Suture reaction	Symmetry	Aesthetic acceptance	Aesthetic acceptance
Suture	Dehiscence	Initial symmetry	Healing	Dyspareunia	Satisfaction
Hematoma	Inflammation	Inflammation	Definitive symmetry	Satisfaction	
Dehiscences	Pain	Pain	Aesthetic acceptance		
Infection	Infection		Dyspareunia		
Pain					

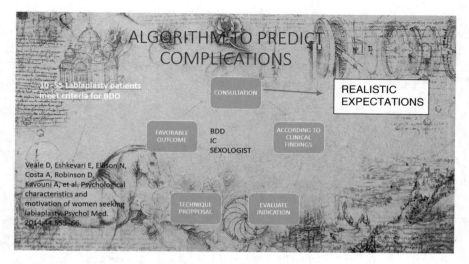

Fig. 10.5 Algorithm to predict complications

At the time of the surgical procedure, the surgeon should follow the guidelines of the topographic labiaplasty; as we know, it allows an adequate approach to all components of a hypertrophy of the labia minora, as well as the presence of anatomical variants, and preserve anatomical repairs, thus the possibility of complications is very low; however I should mention that, when you are starting in the performance of this procedure, the amount of tissue to be resected should be conservative, in order to have the opportunity of an adequate re-intervention in case of being necessary because of aesthetic inconformity from the patient; it must be remembered that "the first cut is the deepest" [8], meaning that we must be careful at the time of performing a labiaplasty, since we not only have in our hands the sexuality of our patients, but we run the risk that this type of procedure can be interpreted as a type of genital mutilation, as stated, for example, by the Canadian Association of Gynecology and Obstetrics to all its associates [9].

Type of Complications

Complications in labiaplasty can occur at different times; they are divided into intraoperative, immediate postoperative, and late.

Intraoperative

We can have an incidental puncture at the moment of the hydrodissection which generates a hematoma; with the use of different energy sources, we can have different degrees of thermal effect, or collateral thermal damage, as previously seen in the corresponding chapter, so that if an inadequate energy is used, the result is carbonization of the tissue, which leads to greater postoperative pain, suture dehiscence, and poor aesthetic results.

The complications described at this time of labiaplasty are strictly related to poor technique, excessive cutting, excessive suture tension, and inappropriate choice of suture material.

Immediate and Immediate Postoperative Period

In this period, the appearance of hematomas is possible; when a proper technique of vascular mapping was not followed, postoperative pain of greater intensity may occur secondary to a hematoma; we can also find early suture dehiscence, within the first 72 h of the procedure and late until day 10; likewise we can find reactions to suture material specifically polyglactin [10]. Finally in this period of the procedure, rarely we can find infections at the surgical site level, in our data this finding has been extremely rare, since we use laser technology, which has bactericidal properties.

Late Complications

The most common late complications are lymphedema, which is usually generated by excessive tension in the suture area, and asymmetry, which can be up to 15%; abnormal scarring and aesthetic discomfort are also aspects that can occur late, and are avoidable, if we follow the guidelines of topographic labiaplasty (Fig. 10.6).

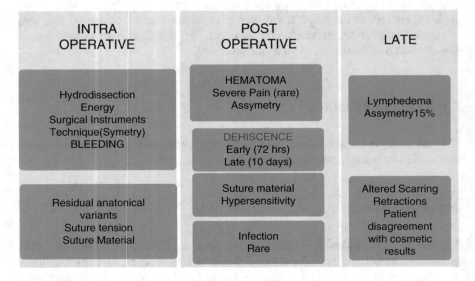

Fig. 10.6 Timing of labiaplasty complications

Miscellaneous Cases of Complications

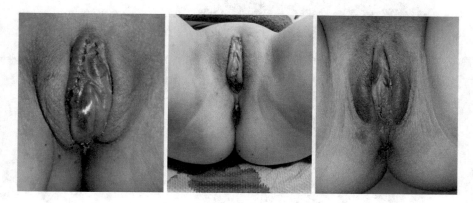

1. Hematomas

   Inadequate cut, invasion of the safety margin of the third compartment (interlabial fold, insertion base of the labia minora concept of topographical labiaplasty

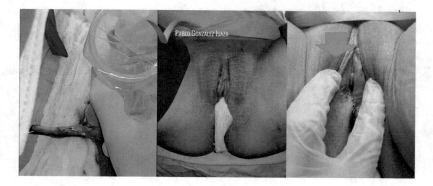

2. Inadequate cutting safety remarks invasion (third compartment) interlabial fold base of insertion of labia minora (topographic labiaplasty concept).

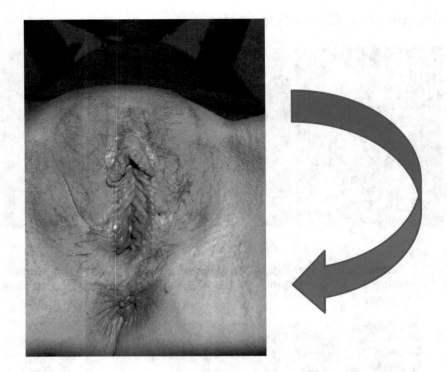

3. Amputations improper cut, invasion of safety margin of compartment 2 (frenulum/insertion complex).

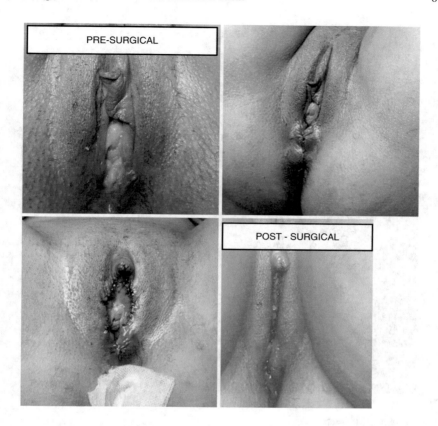

Amputations, safety margin invasion of all topographic labiaplasty compart-
ments (clitoral hood, interlabial fold, frenulum complex and its insertions,
insertion base of the labium). (Courtesy: Dr. Alvaro Ochoa Urogynecologist
Cucuta Colombia).

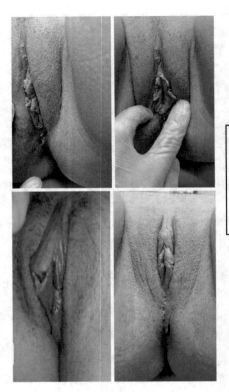

SUTURE DEHISCENCE CAUSES

- Inadequate energy source
- Inadequate Technique
- Excess of suture tension
- Inadequate selection of suture material
- Inadequate vascular mapping

4. Suture dehiscence

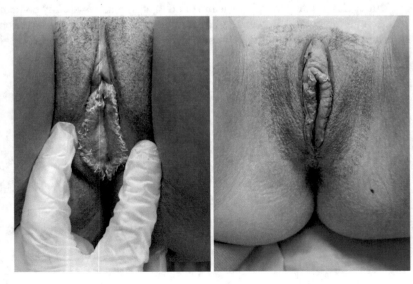

5. Reaction to suture material (polyglactin)

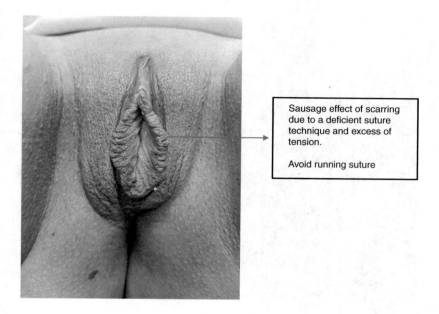

Sausage effect of scarring
due to a deficient suture
technique and excess of
tension.

Avoid running suture

6. Abnormal scarring

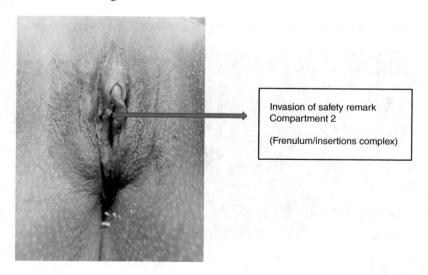

Invasion of safety remark
Compartment 2

(Frenulum/insertions complex)

7. Complications due to lack of knowledge of anatomical repairs and safety remarks

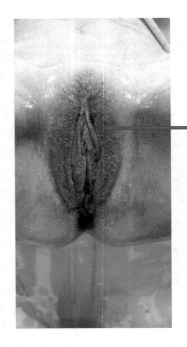

BOTCHED LABIAPLASTY

Non previous approach of
clitoral hood and anatomical
variants in the horizontal plane
(duplications and bifurcations)

Poor Aesthetic result.

8. Complications due to lack of knowledge of anatomical variants

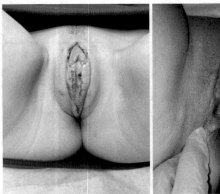

CAUSES OF
LYMPHEDEMA

• No meso
  preservation
• Suture tension
• Bleeding
• Inadequate pop
• Failure to follow
  after care
  recommendations

9. Lymphedema

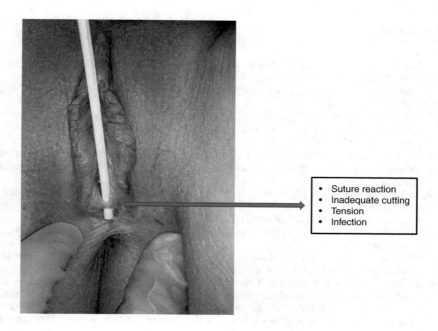

Suture reaction
Inadequate cutting
Tension
Infection

10. Synechiae

Annex 1: Points to Be Included Inside the Informed Consent

Consecutive number
Name of center
Patient ID
Detailed description of the procedure
Smoking history
General risks
Possible complications/indications (aesthetic/functional)
Aesthetic complaints
Revision surgery possibility/second look surgery
Sexual aspects
Downtime
Photos
Videos
Intended uses of videos and photos
Signature best if a witness is present
Companion of patient

References

1. Hamori CA. Postoperative clitoral hood deformity after labiaplasty. Aesthet Surg J. 2013;33(7):1030–6. https://doi.org/10.1177/1090820X13502202.
2. Willis RN, Wong CS, Patel BC. Labiaplasty labia minora reduction. Treasure Island, FL: StatPearls Publishing; 2020.
3. Mirzabeigi MN, Moore JH Jr, Mericli AF, et al. Current trends in vaginal labioplasty: a survey of plastic surgeons. Ann Plast Surg. 2012;68(2):125–34. https://doi.org/10.1097/SAP.0b013e31820d6867.
4. Bucknor A, Chen AD, Egeler S, et al. Labiaplasty: indications and predictors of postoperative sequelae in 451 consecutive cases. Aesthet Surg J. 2018;38(6):644–53. https://doi.org/10.1093/asj/sjx241.
5. Smarrito S, Brambilla M, Berreni N, Paniel BJ. Secondary labiaplasty: retrospective study about 44 cases. Annual report SOFCPRE 2019 Ann Chir Plast Esthet. 2019. pii: S0294-1260(19)30090-1. doi: https://doi.org/10.1016/j.anplas.2019.06.002.
6. Gowda et al. Indications, techniques and complications of labiaplasty. Interesting case. 2015. www.ePlasty.com.
7. Veale D, Eshkevari E, Ellison N, Costa A, Robinson D, Kavouni A, et al. Psychological characteristics and motivation of women seeking labiaplasty. Psychol Med. 2014;44:555–66.
8. Barbara G, Facchin F, Meschia M, Vercellini P. "The first cut is the deepest": a psychological, sexological and gynecological perspective on female genital cosmetic surgery. Acta Obstet Gynecol Scand. 2015;94(9):915–20. https://doi.org/10.1111/aogs.12660. The title caption, "The first cut is the deepest", is a quote from Cat Stevens. In: New Masters. U.K., Decca Records, 1967
9. Shaw D, Lefebvre G, Bouchard C, et al. Female genital cosmetic surgery. J Obstet Gynaecol Can. 2013;35(12):1108–12. https://doi.org/10.1016/S1701-2163(15)30762-3.
10. Cartmill BT, Parham DM, Strike PW, Griffiths L, Parkin B. How do absorbable sutures absorb? A prospective double-blind randomized clinical study of tissue reaction to polyglactin 910 sutures in human skin. Orbit. 2014;33(6):437–43. https://doi.org/10.3109/01676830.2014.950285.

Chapter 11
Secondary Labiaminoraplasty

Massimiliano Brambilla

Introduction

Labia minora reconstruction is a challenging procedure both from the aesthetic and the surgical viewpoint. The increased number of labia reduction and increased number of secondary procedures are encouraging gynecoplasty surgeons to find new techniques such as tissue regenerative procedure in order to increase success.

Preoperative Evaluation

Before the procedure, it is mandatory to define the following:

1. General aesthetic of the vulva, labia minora, and labia majora
2. The technique used in primary surgery
3. The blood flow of labia minora, prepuce, and vulva
4. The quality of the scars
5. The pain and eventual trigger points
6. The patient desires and expectations (according to possibilities and limits)

During the consultation, it is very useful to show to the patient the images of her vulva on a monitor (or at least on a mirror) explaining her residual anatomy and the possible treatments.

Is advisable to tape record the consultation and to sign a personal specific informed consent.

M. Brambilla (✉)
Unit of Plastic and Reconstructive Gynecology, Mangiagalli Hospital, Milan, Italy
e-mail: dr@massimilianobrambilla.it

© The Author(s), under exclusive license to Springer Nature
Switzerland AG 2023
P. Gonzalez-Isaza, R. Sánchez-Borrego (eds.), *Topographic Labiaplasty*,
https://doi.org/10.1007/978-3-031-15048-7_11

Classification of Labia Minora Defects

Labia minora defects may be classified as follows:

1. Defects in excess
2. Defects in defect
3. Skin irregularities
4. Modified pigmentation

Abundant Labia Minora Following Labiareduction

Abundancy may be classified as follows:

1. Partial labia minora abundancy
2. Total labia minora abundancy

1. Monolateral
2. Bilateral

1. Confined to labia minora
2. Extended to the prepuce

Secondary reduction of abundant labia minora following a previous labiaplasty will take into consideration labia minora blood flow and general aesthetic of labia minora.

Excessive Labia Minora Reduction

Defects may be classified as follows:

1. Partial defect of inferior, central, or superior labia minora
2. Total loss of entire labia minora

1. Monolateral
2. Bilateral

Surgical Correction (Figs. 11.1, 11.2, 11.3, 11.4, 11.5, 11.6, 11.7, 11.8, 11.9, 11.10, 11.11, 11.12, 11.13, 11.14, and 11.15)

Regenerative Treatments

Tissue regeneration helps to strengthen the residual labial tissues and perilabial tissues, increasing the possibility of success of secondary procedures.

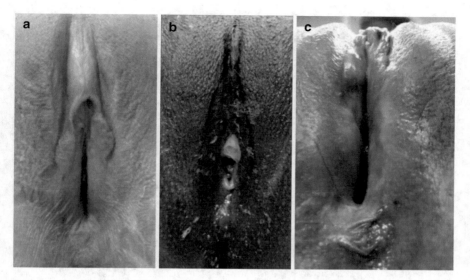

Fig. 11.1 Different etiology, same result (**a**) lichen sclerosus (**b**) female genital mutilation (**c**) aggressive labiaminoraplasty

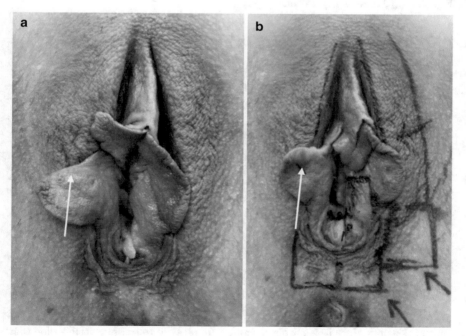

Fig. 11.2 Right labia minora dehiscence postcentral wedge resection. (**a**) Before microfatgraft of the labial margins (arrow on the margin). (**b**) Three months after microfatgraft of the labial margins (arrow on the margin); surgical plan is shown: on the right secondary wedge reconstruction, on the left superiorly based flap inferior transposition labiaplasty and labia majora microfatgraft

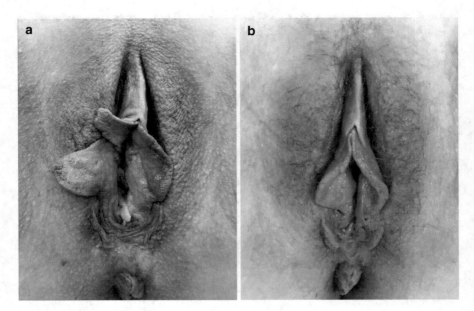

Fig. 11.3 (**a**) Before surgery; (**b**) after surgery

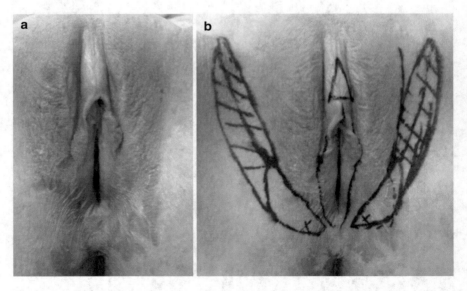

Fig. 11.4 (**a**) Vulvar lichen sclerosus, partial loss of labia minora. (**b**) Surgical plan: micro-/nano-fatgraft, skin graft of the labia minora reconstruction, posterior commissure amplification with perineal flaps

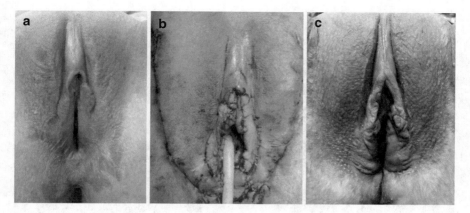

Fig. 11.5 (**a**) Before surgery; (**b**) at 6 days post-op; (**c**) at 2 years post-surgery

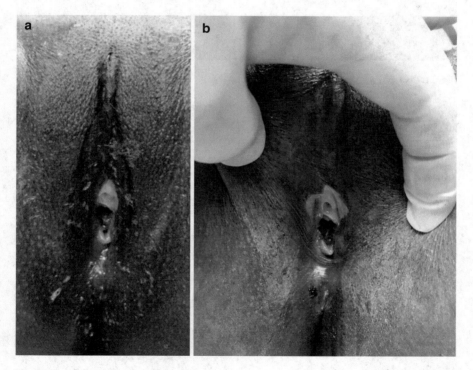

Fig. 11.6 (**a**) FGM type 2 (**b**) posterior commissure stenosis. Surgical plan micro-/nanofatgraft, rigottomies, skin graft labia minora reconstruction

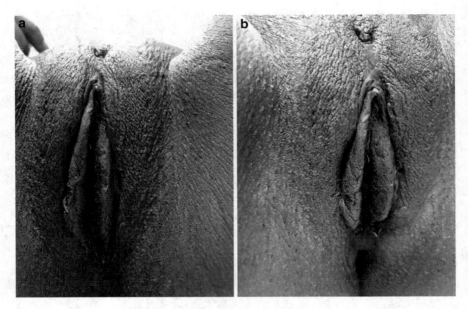

Fig. 11.7 (**a, b**) At 1 year post-op, lateral view

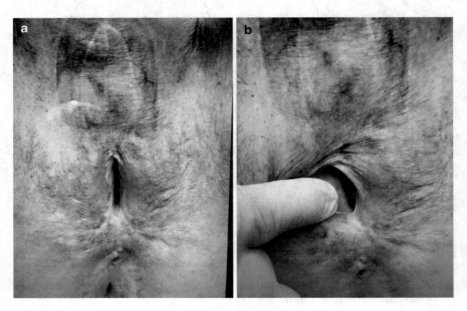

Fig. 11.8 (**a**) Severe lichen vulvar lichen sclerosus with stenosis and postsurgical scars; (**b**) vulvar stenosis

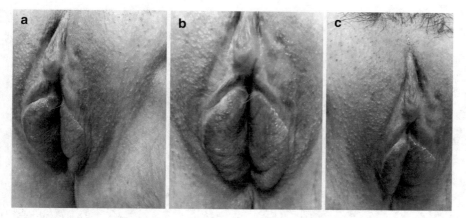

Fig. 11.9 (**a–c**) Post-op at 2 years

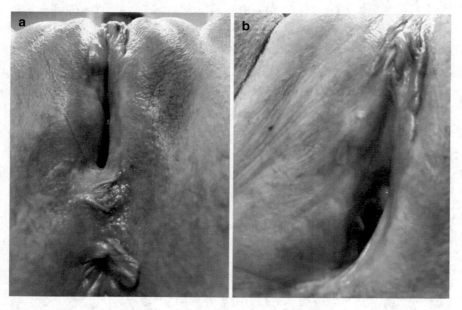

Fig. 11.10 (**a**) Labia minora amputation following labiaminoraplasty; (**b**) posterior commissure stenosis

Microfatgraft procedure: Donor site is infiltrated with a solution of 100 cc saline, 0.25 mL adrenaline, and 20 mg of lidocaine; fat is harvested with a 2 mm multihole cannula and decanted for 10 min or centrifuged for 2 min at 3000 rpm.

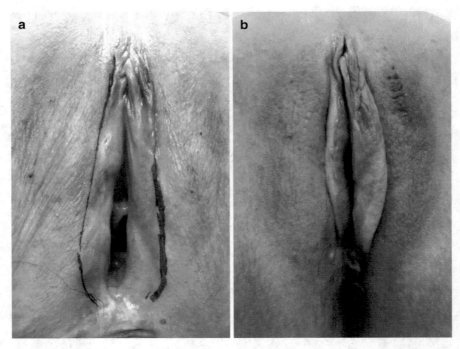

Fig. 11.11 (**a**) Surgical plan: full thickness skin graft reconstruction and micro-/nanofatgraft; (**b**) post-op at 2 years

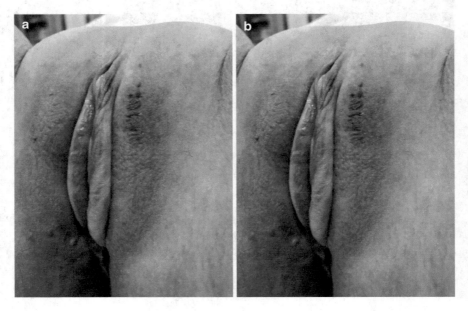

Fig. 11.12 (**a, b**) Post-op at 2 years

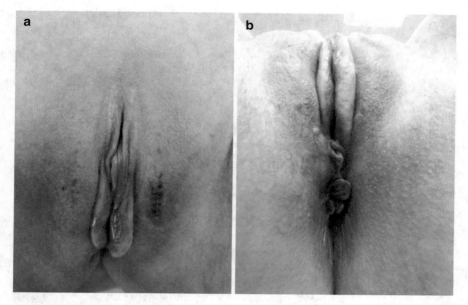

Fig. 11.13 (**a, b**) Post-op at 2 years

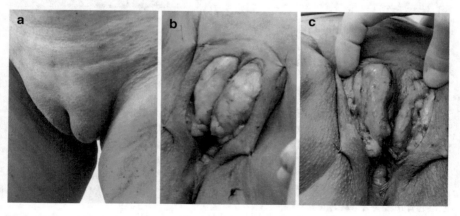

Fig. 11.14 (**a**) Excessive labia minora reduction and excessive labia majora augmentation; (**b**) labia majora dissection; (**c**) left labia majora reduction

0.3/1 mL of microfatgraft is carefully grafted in the residual labia minora and in the scar tissue with an 18-gauge sharp needle.

Two to four months following regenerative injections are needed before surgical correction of the labia minora.

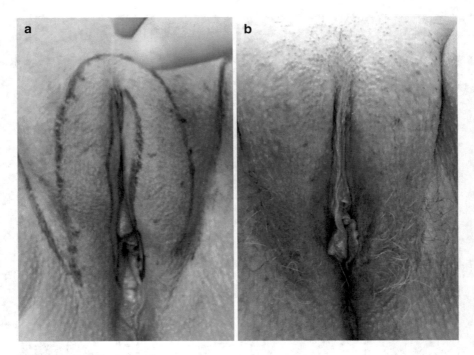

Fig. 11.15 (**a, b**) Post-op at 2 years

Reconstruction of Labia Minora

1. Skin irregularities

    Labia minora margin irregularities may appear on the labia crest as indentations, due to suture marks (to avoid this problem the removal of all sutures is advisable within 10 days from surgery) or due to limited marginal dehiscence [1].

    Indented margin marks can be successfully treated by CO_2 laser resurfacing, while partial resection of the margins and secondary suture is indicated for limited marginal dehiscence.

2. Partial defect inferior to 1/3

    The correction is carried out by excision of 1/2 mm of the margins, and then margins are sutured in a triple plane: neurovascular bundle fixation with 4/0 or 5/0 vycril (according to tissue quality) followed by medial and lateral skin flaps in 5/0 vycril. It is advisable to enhance tissue vascularity injecting PRP or ultrananofatgraft on the margins (0.5 cc per 5 cm).

    NB: The suture of early flaps diastasis is burdened by high risk of dehiscence and is advisable to postpone it at 3 months. If this procedure has to be performed due to "psychological pressure," it is advisable to inject the margins with PRP or ultrananofatgraft in order to reduce inflammation and enhance tissue quality.

3. Partial defect superior to 1/3

   (a) If the defect is superiorly located and prepuce is abundant and intact, an inferiorly based preputial flap may be harvested, transposed inferiorly, and sutured to the residual labia minora [2].
   (b) If the defect is inferiorly located, an inferior flap superiorly based may be superiorly rotated and sutured to the residual labia minora.

      Another option is offered by the two stages procedure. The controlateral labia minora inferiorly or superiorly vascularized is dissected, tubed, and transposed to the defect. After 2–3 weeks, the flap is separated and both labia are reshaped.

4. Total loss of labia minora

   Total loss of labia minora may be due to pathologies such as lichen sclerosus, excessive surgical resection, or FGM. Outcomes are similar with very different etiology.

   (a) Recruiting technique: The residual medial flap is dissected medially and elevated 2/3 cm, the lateral flap is sutured with multiple 5/0 vycril at the base of the flap, and the margins are sutured together. This may allow a 1.5/2 cm labia reconstruction [3, 4].
   (b) Full thickness skin graft reconstruction: An incision 1.5 cm lateral to the original scar, including the scar itself, is carried out. The flap is elevated with 0.2/0.3 cm subdermal thickness in order to grant optimal vascularity. A full thickness skin graft is harvested from the inguinal or gluteal crease; the dimension of the graft varies according to the defect to be covered. The skin graft is fixed to the medial labial flap with 5/0 vycril, and a compression is held in place for 5 days as well as the catheter. To enhance tissue vascularity and reduce inflammatory reactions, PRP or ultrananofatgraft is injected into the margins (0.5 cc per 5 cm).

      In order to enhance skin graft quality and elasticity, nanofat graft is injected under the dermis 3 months after the procedure.
   (c) Double tunneled labia majora flap is very useful in case of severe vulvar stenosis and loss of labia minora. The flaps based on the fat pad are harvested and tunneled medially. The reconstruction is very successful from the functional point of view, while from the aesthetic viewpoint, the two tunneled flaps resemble labia minora.
   (d) Ancillary procedures: If labia majora are excessively abundant, their reduction may be optically helpful, enhancing the protrusion.

References

1. ISAPS. Labiaplasty: year-to-year comparisons. 2016. https://www.isaps.org/wp-content/uploads/2017/10/GlobalStatistics2016-1.pdf.

2. Alter GJ. Labia minora reconstruction using clitoral hood flaps, wedge excisions and YV advancement flaps. Plast Reconstr Surg. 2011;127(6):2356–63.
3. Gress S. Labia minora repair. Aesthet Plast Surg. 2022;45:2447–63.
4. O'Dey DM. Complex vulvar reconstruction following female genital mutilation/cutting. Urologe A. 2017;56(10):1298–301.

Chapter 12
Labiaplasty in Adolescents

Maryory Gomez

In recent years we have seen articles in magazines, where they strongly criticize the increase of labiaplasty in adolescents, generating concern both in the social environment and in the scientific community. Recent data reports a 50% increase from 1 year to another and with statistics that are on the rise especially with the aim for aesthetic improvement. A research in the United Kingdom showed in 2010 an increase of five times the number of surgeries compared to the previous 10 years. From 2008 to 2012 in the UK, the National Health Service recorded 297 labiaplasty in girls under the age of 14 [1].

In social magazines we see headlines like this one in Argentina *more and more teenagers are having genital surgery in Rosario* [2] or like this one from Mexico which refers to *labiaplasty as a sad genital plastic surgery that is growing in popularity among teenagers* [3]. An American publication that describes that labiaplasty in adolescents is on the rise as a concern of teenagers for their appearance and symmetry [4], and finally a Spanish article *The labiaplasty the latest fashion trend among young women* which reflects a study where they measured different vulvas; they visualized a significant variety of vulvar anatomy, not finding the concept of what can be a normal vulva; Australia reports that girls as young as 9 years old were undergoing this procedure because of misinformation and insecurities about the appearance of their genitalia [5].

The concern is not only at the level of social magazines but also in scientific journals such as the one published by Bragagnini Rodriguez and collaborators in 2015 *Hypertrophy of labia minora, a growing problem in adolescence* [4].

This increase may be related to the fact that nowadays teenagers have easier access to images of idealized female genitalia, generating anxiety about how individual anatomy should be; they even have access to images that might have been

M. Gomez (✉)
Dr. Rafael Guerra Méndez Clinical Centre, Valencia, Venezuela
e-mail: dragomez@ginecoestetica.com

105

retouched or models that may represent the real appearance of few women, to this is added the use of a complete hair removal that allows them to detail their vulva [6]; this can lead a teenager to feel confused and believe that a surgery is needed.

But the concern does not end in the increase of these surgeries but who are performing them, how are they performed, and if it is really justified to perform this surgery at this age; in my experience, I have had cases where malpractice has been practiced, wrongly called complications. That is why it is important to mention that this type of patients has the risk of reaching untrained hands that can cause great physical and psychological damage.

Thus, it is important to describe four important elements for the successful practice of labia minora labiaplasty in this age group.

When to Perform Labiaplasty in Adolescents?

It is important to remember some aspects about the development of this stage called adolescence, where its beginning and progression vary with a wide range of normality, allowing us to establish criteria for the performance of labiaplasty. In terms of concepts we have that puberty includes organic changes, being the most noticeable, and the development of secondary sexual characteristics, while adolescence encompasses physical, psychological, emotional, and social changes [7].

The World Health Organization divides adolescence into two stages: first adolescence (10–14 years) and second adolescence (15–19 years), this classification being based on chronology. However, the American Society for Adolescent Health and Medicine (SAHM) places adolescence between 10 and 21 years, as it includes psychosocial development, distinguishing three phases that overlap each other:

1. Early adolescence from 10 to 13 years of age and is characterized primarily by pubertal changes.
2. Middle adolescence, ages 14–17, is a time when risky behaviors can begin.
3. Late adolescence or youth, from the age of 18–21 years old, in which important physical growth and development are achieved and the psychosocial objectives necessary for the evolution of the young person to adulthood are reached [8, 9].

Physical Development

From the age of 15 years, girls have reached sexual maturity; at this age they have passed the stage of puberty, so we will focus between middle and late adolescence. With respect to the hormonal axis, it includes both the regularity of menstrual cycles and the influence on the development of different parts of the body, through mainly estrogenic stimuli so that the presence of the feminine sexual characteristics takes place. The vulvar area also receives important stimuli by the presence of both estrogenic and androgenic receptors, reaching maturity this axis at 3 years after menarche.

From the point of view of their maturation process, physical growth is initially disharmonious, growing in segments until they achieve full development, reaching an adult body with redistribution of body fat. Each person comes to have a pattern of development, the earlier the age of onset of puberty, the greater the gain in size during puberty, so that females can reach their final size between 16 and 17 years [6–8].

With the beginning of estrogen secretion by the ovary, the vulva begins to have a stimulated appearance: the labia majora and minora increase in volume, pigmentation of the labia minora, the size of the hymen increases, and genital discharge begins to appear. When puberty is complete, the growth of the labia majora and minora ends, and the clitoris can already be identified as an erectile organ [10].

Chronological age has little correlation with sexual maturity, and growth can be highly variable. A guide for us is the index of sexual maturation which is assessed by Tanner's stages (1962) which is based on the development of the genital organs and secondary sexual characteristics. So to know that this adolescent has reached the right proportion of her body, she should be in Tanner stages 3–4, since the maximum speed of growth occurs between these stages, coinciding with an average age between 14 and 16 years [7–9].

Cognitive and Moral Development

- In middle adolescence they believe that everyone is looking out for their behaviors or appearance.
- They think they are unique and special.
- They are able to reflect and distinguish between truth and falsehood.
- Feelings of omnipotence and immortality: risky behaviors.
- They are searching for their identity.
- They look for role models in leaders; they are interested above all in the present.
- After the age of 17, they have the capacity for analysis and reflection; they see beyond their own reality; they are more concerned about their future and have a rational and realistic conscience.
- Concretization of moral, religious, and sexual values [6, 7, 11].

Emotional Development

- In middle adolescence they think about themselves, worry about their appearance, and feel insecure about their attractiveness.
- Fashion and advertising lead them to admire a particular body stereotype.
- They lack the maturity to control their reaction when they have a setback.

- They have oppositional or negativistic behaviors.
- In late adolescence they are more independent and more emotionally stable.
- They don't feel like victims and have a very clear identity.
- They place more value on their own image, and some are happy with the way they look.
- Worries disappear [6, 7, 11].

So, if we know when teenagers reach maturity in their development, not only physically, psychologically, but also cognitively, morally, and emotionally, we can establish criteria to perform labia minora labiaplasty on the adolescent population:

1. Remember that not everyone reaches maturity at the same time. Conservative medical treatment should be tried first, recommending the use of loose clothing and good genital hygiene, in such a way as to bring it to the age at which we believe that labia growth has reached its limit [7, 11, 12].
2. Do not perform this type of surgery in the absence of menarche or without formed sexual characteristics, so it is important to take as a guide to sexual maturity Tanner stages and wait until they are in stages 3–4 [7, 8, 10, 11].
3. This should be done 3–4 years after menarche, making sure not only that there is sufficient sexual maturity but also psychological and emotional maturity. This will give us an approximate age between 15 and 16 years, taking an average menarche of 11–12 years; of course it will depend on the pattern they have in each of the countries [13].
4. Patients with associated symptoms. It is one of the criteria that becomes more relevant, even more than the size of the labia minora is the degree of discomfort for functional, psychological, and aesthetic reasons [1, 13–15].
5. Perform labiaplasty considering hypertrophy in labia greater than 4 cm or type 3 according to Motakef's classification [14–16].
6. Be careful in patients who present asymmetry even if they are described in 17–25%, as it has already been explained that during these 4 years after menarche, there are also hormonal receptors in the vulva that can continue to stimulate the unequal growth of both labia [6, 17].
7. If the adolescent desires surgery, she must express specific concerns and have realistic goals, must show maturity and understand the procedure, the risks, and consequences, and should not initiate the request for surgery on behalf of the parents. The American Society of Plastic Surgery demonstrated that surgical procedures resulting from the personal demands of the adolescent have a more favorable outcome than when they begin with the perceptions of their family [1, 6].
8. Where distress is considered significant, psychological assessment should be sought [6, 12].
9. Body dysmorphic disorder. We cannot forget to rule it out in the evaluation [18]. What is important to know is that there are publications or works such as Springgs M, Gilliam L. **Body Dysmorphic Disorder: Contraindication or Ethical Justification for female genital cosmetics surgery in adolescents** where they show that improving a part of the body that can cause them concern

generates a better quality of life, but of course you have to know how to choose. They question those who claim that there would be no benefit from surgery in this situation and consider the possible harm that could be caused if treatment is refused in this type of patient [19].

10. The British Society for pediatric and adolescent gynecology considers that there is no enough scientific evidence to support the practice of labiaplasty, for girls under the age of 18 years, counseling should be the most convenient approach, and labiaplasty should be the last resource [20].

Finally, in May 2016 the American College of Obstetrics and Gynecology (ACOG) publishes recommendations about labia surgery in adolescents [18].

- When adolescent girls seek medical treatment, the first step should be education and reassurance regarding normal variation in anatomy, growth, and development.
- Appropriate counseling and assessment of physical maturity and emotional readiness are necessary prior to surgical treatment or referral.
- Adolescent girls should be screened for body dysmorphic disorder if deemed appropriate by the gynecologist.
- The obstetrician-gynecologist caring for the adolescent should have a good working knowledge for comfort and appearance, as well as knowledge of the indications and timing of surgical intervention and referral.

They also describe that adolescent girls often wish to improve physical conditions that they perceive as defective and if left uncorrected can affect them into adulthood. This age group may be under particular stress with regard to these problems because of societal conceptions of the ideal female body and parental concerns about bodily perfection. Although reconstructive procedures aimed at correcting abnormalities (caused by congenital defects, trauma, infection, or disease) or cosmetic procedures performed to reshape normal structures may improve function, appearance, and self-esteem, not all adolescents are suitable for surgical intervention.

How to Assess the Adolescent?

The environment in which the examination is performed is fundamental. Privacy and comfort are mandatory rules for this type of examination.

The most important thing is to establish a good doctor-patient relationship that eliminates the fear of gynecological exploration and allows the answer to the questions they want to raise. Among the causes for which these young women seek this type of surgery are usually described: local irritation, discomfort when walking or sitting, hygiene problems and fissures during menstruation, discomfort when playing sports, volume increase, or aesthetics.

As for the companion will depend on the age of the teenager in conjunction with the laws governing in each country, it is usually left to choose the teenager if they can be or not their parents mainly her mother; however, for the evaluation of this surgery before 18 years of age, it is suggested that the doctor reserves a time alone with the girl to inquire about their real needs, but in turn it is advisable that they are accompanied for the understanding of the procedure if it applies according to the criteria.

The examination to be performed varies depending on whether or not she has had penetrative sexual intercourse. If she has not had intercourse, an inspection of the external genitalia is performed in the butterfly or frog position (Fig. 12.1). With lateral traction maneuvers of the labia majora (Fig. 12.2), and if she has had penetrative intercourse, the examination will be performed in the lithotomy position [10, 21]. It is important for the adolescent's peace of mind to explain each action before

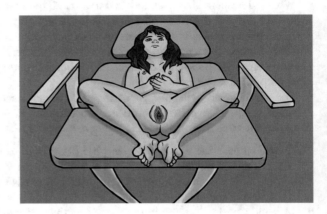

Fig. 12.1 Butterfly position

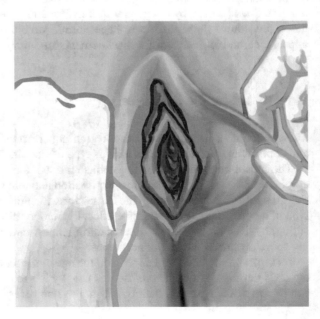

Fig. 12.2 Traction of labia minora

performing it, and it is also essential that the patient and the doctor view the genitalia simultaneously using a colposcope or mirror, in order to explain the anatomy, and understand it and the type of technique to be performed if surgery is considered.

Finally, once the adolescent has been fully evaluated and has accepted the conditions of the surgery, an informed consent form must be signed by both the adolescent and one of her companions [22].

Selection of Technique

To choose the appropriate technique at this age should be taken into consideration: the one that is less complex but is also appropriate according to the anatomy of the labia minora, with low rate of complications such as suture dehiscence, which does not require excessive care as they are restless patients who may not comply with the post operative indications and of course the technique that dominates the surgeon. Likewise, it should take importance to perform a clitoral hood reduction if necessary as this may be a reason for a reintervention in the future.

This type of surgery is not only based on choosing the technique and seeing the vulva in a plane, but it presents different dimensions and proportions allowing to find the adequate harmonization of this area, starting from the gold standard. Therefore, when evaluating the length of the labia minora identified as "b" and the vulvar fourchette or posterior commissure identified as "d," it is imperative to also visualize the clitoral hood identified as "a" since it is the guiding point together with point "c" for the harmonization of the middle part of the vulva (Fig. 12.3).

Fig. 12.3 Photo showing the points to be considered for the harmonization of the area. (**a**) Clitoral hood, (**b**) Labia minora, (**c**) Glans clitoris, (**d**) The vulvar fourchette or posterior commissure

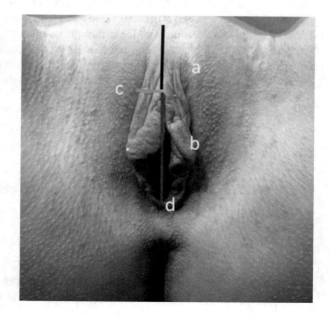

When considering the surgical technique in this age group, the most used are the simple incision and the wedge technique either in its middle part known as alter technique or in its lower edge. As for complications, those described in the publications range from 2% to 5% related to dehiscence, reporting in most cases satisfactory results [1, 12–15, 20, 23–25].

P.K. Jotilakshmi and collaborators in the United Kingdom, **Labial reduction in adolescent population: a case series study**, published in 2009, already spoke of the popularity of labia minora reduction in adolescents. The sample consisted of six patients aged 11–16 years, two with mental health problems who were offered psychological help, three with bilateral reduction, and three with unilateral reduction; the techniques used were simple incision and wedge, without complications and a follow-up of only 3 months [26].

P. Bragagnini et al. at the Miguel Servet Children's Hospital, Zaragoza, **Labia minora hypertrophy, a growing problem in adolescence**, in 2015. With a sample of 29 patients, the age was between 11 and 15 years, 16 with surgery criteria. With simple incision technique, one recurrence of one of the labia and the median follow-up time was 1 year [23].

Yarumi Ochoa Gilbert and collaborators of the Cerro Pediatric Teaching Hospital, Havana, Cuba, **Hypertrophy of labia minora at puberty** published in 2018, conducted a descriptive study of 21 patients, with an average age of 13 years (11–14 years); the technique used was simple distal edge resection; 76.2% was bilateral; they required clitoral hood surgery 14.3%; one complication was reported. The results of the surgical technique used were aesthetically and functionally satisfactory [20].

In my experience for over 10 years working in the area of cosmetic gynecology, between May 2017 and September 2018, reduction labiaplasty was performed on 25 patients, 7 in ages between 10 and 16 years and 18 in ages between 17 and 21 years. There were no complications and the technique used was single incision, and out of those 25 patients, 13 patients required clitoral hood reduction. The first reason for surgery was discomfort with tight clothing in 100%, second reason with 84% was the presence of fissures in the vulvar area during menstruation, and 72% in third place for aesthetic reasons.

Complications

Complications in different works range from 2% to 5% have been described:

- Bruising
- Edema
- Infections
- Dehiscence

Regarding dehiscence, it is the most frequent and it is related with the type of technique, especially wedge techniques [27], such as the one shown in the image

Fig. 12.4 Dehiscence of the insertion at the base of both labia after performing wedge technique

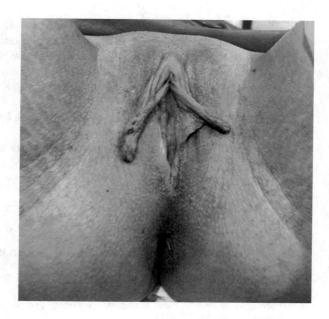

(Fig. 12.4). Orange et al. describe 10% wound dehiscence in cases using wedge resection and hematomas in 40% with a Z-plasty technique.

Oranges et al. conducted a review of the literature on surgical techniques that included 38 studies published between 1971 and 2014, involving 1981 patients as young as 10 years of age, with the most common complications being wound dehiscence, hematoma formation, postoperative bleeding, and urinary retention. All studies reported a satisfaction rate of over 90% and a complication rate of 6.76%; none considered serious; also important is the effect of changing practice over the years and different surgical techniques. The author also cites a revision surgery rate of 1.7% linked to the perception that insufficient tissue had been removed [28].

Since there may be a labia minora growth due to factors such as hormonal stimulation, situations such as pregnancy, fibroepithelial changes due to the constant rubbing of the area, among others; sometimes the permanence of the result of the surgery cannot be assured, and this is relevant to be discussed with adolescents.

Conclusions

- The British Society for pediatric and adolescent gynecology considers that there is no enough scientific evidence to support the practice of labiaplasty; for girls under the age of 18 years, counseling should be the most convenient approach, and labiaplasty should be the last resource.
- First there must be a counseling about the anatomy of the vulva, before deciding any surgical procedure. Sometimes they come to the consultation asking for

guidance as to whether what they are feeling or seeing is abnormal. Therefore, during the first evaluation visit, it is essential to be clear about what should be examined and the emphasis that the adolescent may express in terms of her symptoms.

- Considering the different criteria reduces complications and avoids any functional or psychological damage.
- The technique to be applied must be selected for each case, easy to perform, and with low risk of complications.
- Labiaplasty in adolescents should be performed by trained and experienced surgeons.

References

1. Battisti C, Milanesi ML, De Freitas NF, Krauterbluth P, Junior S, Bins P. Treatment of hypertrophy of small vaginal lips in adolescence - current experience of the Hospital da Criança Santo Antônio da Santa Casa de Misericórdia de Porto Alegre. Rev Bras Cir Plást. 2018;33(Suppl. 1):175–7.
2. Ferrarece S. More and more teenagers are having genital surgery in Rosario. Rosario, Argentina, December 14, 2017.
3. https://www.rosario3.com/noticias/Cada-vez-mas-adolescentes-se-operan-los-genitales-en-Rosario-20171213-0027.html.
4. Osborne S. Teen labioplasty surgery is on the rise as teenagers worry about appearance and symmetry, United Kingdom, 28 April 2016. https://www.independent.co.uk/news/world/americas/teen-labiaplasty-surgery-is-on-the-rise-as-adolescents-worry-about-appearance-and-symmetry-a7006081.html.
5. Ander A. Lip plasty the latest "pussy" fashion craze in young girls, 18 July 2018, Spain.
6. Boraei S, Clark C, Frith L. Labioplasty in girls under 18 years of age: an unethical procedure. Clin Ethics. 2008;3:37–41.
7. Güemes-Hidalgo M, Ceñal GM, Hidalgo VM. Pubertad y Adolescencia. Adolescere. 2017;V(1):7–22.
8. Casas JJ, Ceñal MJ. Adolescent development. Physical, psychological and social aspects. Pediatr Integral. 2005;9:20–4.
9. Castellano G, Hidalgo MI, Redondo AM. Adolescent medicine. Comprehensive care. Madrid: Ergon; 2004.
10. Parera N, De Alvarez SM, Calaf AJ, Ros RR, Cornellá CJ. Clinical manifestations of puberty in males and females. Manual de Salud Reproductiva. 3:101–51. https://ccp.ucr.ac.cr/bvp/pdf/manual/saludreproductiva/03%20Salud%20reproductiva%20e.pdf
11. Yglesias DJ. Adolescent development: physical, psychological and social aspects. Pediatr Integral. 2013;XVII(2):88–93.
12. Wood P. Cosmetic general surgery in children and adolescents. Clin Obstet Gynaecol. 2018;48:137–46.
13. Reddy J, Laufer RM. Hypertrophyc Labia minora. Mini review. J Pediatr Adolesc Gynecol. 2010;23:3–6.
14. Rodriguez S, Torres A, Enriquez E, Ayuso R, Santamaria JI. Hypertrophy of labia minora in puberty. Cir Pediatr. 2009;22:109–11.
15. Monteagudo BM, Monteagudo L, Yglesias YA. Labia minora hypertrophy in an adolescent girl. Presentation of a patient, Hospital Ginecoobstetrico Universitario "Mariana Grajales", Medigraphic; 2012.

16. Hamori C, Banwell P, Alinsod R. Female cosmetic genital surgery. Concepts, classification and techniques. In: Banwell P, editor. Anatomy and classification of the female genitalia: implications for surgical management. New York: Thieme Medical Publishers, inc; 2017. p. 4–22.
17. Hamori C. Teen labioplasty: a response to the May 2016 American College of Obstetricians and Gynecologyst (ACOG) recommendations on labioplasty in adolescents. Aesthet Surg J. 2016;36(7):807–9.
18. Committee Opinion No. 662: Breast and labial surgery in adolescents. Obstet Gynecol. 2016;127(5):e138–40.
19. Spriggs M, Gilliam L. Body dysmorphic disorder: contraindication or ethical justification for female genital cosmetics surgery in adolescents. Bioethics. 2016;30(9):706–13.
20. Ochoa GY, Rodríguez M, Pérez J. Hypertrophy of labia minora in puberty J Urol. 2018;7(1).
21. Gynecological examination in girls and adolescents. https://sego.es/mujeres/Exploracion_ninas.pdf.
22. Arbo A, Ayala F, Irala A. Adolescence clinical manual. Comprehensive management of adolescents with a rights-based approach. Asunción, Paraguay: Ministry of Public Health and Social Welfare; 2012.
23. Bragagnini RP, Alvarez GN, Gonzalez RY, Ruiz TM, Escartin VR, Gonzalez NM. Labia minora hypertrophy. A growing problem in adolescence. Cir Pediatr. 2015;28:196–9.
24. Runacres SA, Wood PL. Cosmetic labioplasty in an adolescent population. J Pediatr Adolesc Gynecol. 2016;29(3):218–22.
25. Lynch A, Marulaiah M, Samarakkody U. Reduction labioplasty in adolescents. J Pediatr Adolesc Gynecol. 2008;21(3):147–9.
26. Jothilakshmi PK, Salvi RN, Hayden BE, Bose-Haider B. Labial reduction in adolescent population - a case series study. J Pediatr Adolesc Gynecol. 2009;22:53–5.
27. Georgiou CA, Venatar M, Dumas P, et al. A cadaveric study of the arterial blood supply of the labia minora. Plast Reconstr Surg. 2015;136:167.
28. Oranges CM, Sisti A, Sisti G. Labia minora reduction techniques. A comprehensive literature review. Aesthet Surg J. 2015;35(4):419–31.

Chapter 13
What Comes After a Labiaplasty

Diana Lorena Velez Rizo

Introduction

Labia minora reduction labiaplasty is a highly requested procedure in which a sufficient resection is sought to preserve an adequate and harmonious external genital anatomy, respecting the functionality and neurovascular structures for a better postoperative result.

In the literature, studies report a maximum follow-up of 6 years with frequent loss of patients in the study population, a phenomenon mainly explained by the high rate of satisfaction with the procedure.

More than half of women tend not to talk about their discomfort to their relatives, friends, or parents about the size of labia minora; complaints can be either functional, aesthetic, or sexual. This scenario changes drastically in the postsurgical state where more than 95% of women recommend the procedure and manifest a positive change in their lives that improves their self-esteem [1].

To evaluate the results and changes after labiaplasty, it is important to know the motivations and expectations of women before undergoing the surgical procedure. It has been described that 71% of women express concern about their appearance, 61% physical discomfort symptoms, 31% emotional concern with sexual relations, and 17.4% general discomfort in daily life. Up to 40.4% claim functional causes to the local health system (irritation, discomfort with tight clothing, during physical exercise, with sexual activity, and difficulty with hygiene), but few are covered by these basic health plans [2–4].

In this chapter, we will review the implications and postsurgical events related to labia minora reduction labiaplasty.

D. L. V. Rizo (✉)
Gynecology Department, Dra. Diana Vélez Rizo Ginecología Avanzada - Fundación Cardioinfantil, Bogotá D.C., Cundinamarca, Colombia
e-mail: info@dianavelezginecologa.com

P. Gonzalez-Isaza, R. Sánchez-Borrego (eds.), *Topographic Labiaplasty*, https://doi.org/10.1007/978-3-031-15048-7_13

117

Prognostic Factors for Postoperative Sequelae

Age of Surgical Procedure

It has been described that patients who have undergone labiaplasty at an early age may present again with labia minora hypertrophy since they are still growing under hormonal influences, without determining in the literature an exact percentage of recurrence.

The implications of labiaplasty in adolescence are explored with emphasis on knowledge of normality or perceived normal genital appearance, pubertal development, anatomy, physiology, and options for surgical intervention, including risks and complications.

The recommendations of the *ACOG* (*American College of Obstetricians and Gynecologists*) emphasize the importance of education, counseling, and making appropriate surgical decisions with adolescent patients interested in genital cosmetic surgery, to determine the compromise of quality of life due to hypertrophy of the labia minora, ruling out associated pathologies and thus assessing whether to defer the procedure versus performing it. In case of deciding to take the patient to surgery, it is recommended that it be at least 2 years after menarche [5].

In view of the general recommendations on female cosmetic genital surgery, such interventions should be avoided in adolescence in the absence of definite medical indications until at least 18 years of age [6].

Smoking

Smoking is a well-known risk factor for poor healing that impacts postoperative outcomes. It has been estimated that postoperative complications are more prevalent in female smokers vs. nonsmokers at a ratio of 21% versus 11% [7].

Therefore, the patient should be advised to stop smoking at least 2 months before and 2 months after the procedure in order to improve healing response and reduce the risk of complications.

Female Sexual Dysfunction

Another poor prognostic factor defined in the literature for postoperative labiaplasty is the presence of *female sexual dysfunction* as an indication for surgery, since it increases the need for revision surgery in a statistically significant way (31.3% vs. 10.7%, $P = 0.002$).

Because female sexual dysfunction is of a multifactorial origin, in patients who consider labiaplasty as a solution to this condition an additional assessment to study symptoms related to dysfunction, such as altered phases of sexual response and pain before the procedure, is mandatory to rule out that labia minora hypertrophy is the cause of sexual dysfunction [7].

While labiaplasty has been shown in multiple publications to improve overall sexual satisfaction, it does not mean that it is performed to improve the phases of sexual response (desire, interest, arousal, and orgasm) or for pain that limits sexual intercourse.

Body Dysmorphic Syndrome

The presence of *body dysmorphic syndrome* is identified in 7–13% of people seeking aesthetic treatments.

This should be suspected preoperatively when there is an excessive preoccupation with a defect of mild or unobservable appearance that is associated with obsessive thinking and compulsive behaviors that lead to impact daily living activities [8].

Body dysmorphic syndrome is the most relevant neuropsychiatric condition inside aesthetic procedures where frequently the ideal expectations of patients exceed what is actually achieved with a surgical procedure, and results in greater likelihood of dissatisfaction in the postoperative period; therefore, there is a need to improve the identification of this condition because it usually causes suffering and substantial impairment and limitations [9].

Diagnostic criteria

- Concern about one or more perceived defects or imperfections in physical appearance that are not observable or seem unnoticed by others.
- At some point during the course of the disorder, the subject exhibits obsessive behaviors (e.g., looking in the mirror, excessive grooming, scratching the skin, wanting to make sure of things) or mental acts (e.g., comparing one's appearance to others) that are repetitive in response to worries with appearance.
- The condition causes clinically significant distress or impairment in social, occupational, or other important areas of functioning.
- Concern about appearance is not best explained by the amount fat tissue or body weight in a subject whose symptoms meet diagnostic criteria for an eating disorder.

The use of validated instruments in preoperative evaluations to assess the level of distress regarding physical appearance and satisfaction helps patient selection in a more effective and practical way [10].

The COPS-L scale (*Cosmetic Procedure Screening Scale modified for labia minora labiaplasty*) focuses on concerns about labia minora appearance and is derived from the COPS scale (*Cosmetic Procedure Screening Scale*) that assesses general appearance. COPS-L focuses on the domains of perceived abnormality, effect on sexual relationship, interference with leisure activities, and comparison with others. The questionnaire is answered according to a *Likert* scale ranging from

0 to 8 for each of the questions. It is scored by adding up all the items to provide a total score. The total possible scores range from 0 to 72. Scores above 40 reflect greater alteration, distress, and disability with a body characteristic and, therefore, the likelihood of a diagnosis of *body dysmorphic syndrome* (Annex 1) [11].

Body dysmorphic syndrome is a disorder that can be treated ideally in a multidisciplinary scenario with psychiatry and/or psychology using either pharmacological management and/or cognitive behavioral therapy; the latter has been effective in 2/3 of patients with the disorder with improvement of up to 84.6% [9].

With the abovementioned *body dysmorphic syndrome* is a possible contraindication for an aesthetic procedure. It is recommended in case of clinical suspicion, to apply the detection scale and consider psychological or psychiatric evaluation before giving surgical endorsement.

Early Onset of Postoperative Sexual Activity

Patients who feel that their labia negatively impact their sex life may be more inclined to resume sexual activity very soon after surgery, even earlier than recommended by their surgeon, thereby increasing the risk of dehiscence, bleeding, pain, and early complications [7].

Evaluation

Among the available tools for quantifying satisfaction with genital appearance before and after surgery, the most widely used, is the validated GAS (*Genital Appearance Satisfaction*) scale, which has 11 items on attitudes towards genital appearance. Each item is scored between 0 and 3 (from "never" to "always") with total scores between 0 and 33. The higher the score, the greater the genital dissatisfaction (Annex 2) [11].

Assessing the presence of *female sexual dysfunction* and *body dysmorphic syndrome* with the *Female Sexual Function Index* (FSFI) (Annex 3) and COPS-L scales, respectively, helps to guide medical decisions and the patient in order to clarify expectations, raise awareness, educate, and guide patients [12].

The FSFI was described by Rosen in 2000, it is a 19-item questionnaire with psychometric properties designed to be an instrument for the assessment of female sexual function. It is used to measure sexual function in heterosexual women who have been sexually active in the past 4 weeks. The questions are answered on a *Likert* scale ranging from 0 to 5 or 1 to 5 depending on the item and includes a total of six factors (desire, arousal, lubrication, orgasm, satisfaction, and pain). Total scores less than or equal to 26 indicate the presence of sexual dysfunction [13].

Early and Late Symptoms

In the literature the complication rate varies between 2% and 13% with the overall complication rate in most reports being 4%, and 50% of them refer to the sensation of incomplete resection of the tissue of the labium minora [1].

Early Symptoms

They occur in the early postoperative days, mainly in the first and second week. Up to 13.3% of women report symptoms not related to complications but transiently indicate discomfort that are self-resolved and are related to the procedure such as swelling and pain.

0.2% present immediate complications such as bleeding, 2–6% suture dehiscence. Necrosis and hematomas are described in less than 2%. These complications are avoided and reduced by preserving the anatomical structures and removing only the skin of the labia minora according to the principles of topographical labiaplasty since the vascular and nervous structures are respected [1–7].

Dyspareunia is a symptom described in up to 23% of patients from day 3 post-surgery up to 90 days postoperatively. Ideally one should wait an average of 36 days to resume sexual intercourse regardless of the technique used [14].

Up to 3–6% may require revision labiaplasty which is ideally scheduled after 90 days postoperatively [7].

Depending on the instrument used for the procedure (electroscalpel, laser, radiofrequency, scissors, etc.), in an average of 23 days a woman is ready to return to her normal life [1].

Considering that the multi-pulsed CO_2 laser is gentler with the tissue and has less collateral thermal damage, recovery is faster as it generates more precise cuts, and with less inflammation, patients can return to their daily lives in 3–4 days.

Late Symptoms

Vulvar sensitivity One of the most common criticisms against performing labiaplasty is the dichotomy between loss of sensitivity and hypersensitivity. So far there is no study that confirms these arguments against the procedure, and, in addition, given the volume of procedures performed around the world, it is difficult to determine the exact frequency of each of the techniques used. Kelishadi et al. demonstrated in a cadaveric study the heterogeneity of nerve endings in the labia minora and concluded that because of this it is unlikely that labiaplasty would be related to a loss of sensation [15].

Subsequently, a study was carried out with evaluation of sensitivity to touch before and after labiaplasty with vertical or *edge* technique in combination with clitoral hood plasty. In this study they used criteria of minimum postoperative labia minora length of 1.5 cm from interlabial fold and clitoral hood (from interlabial sulcus to most prominent position) with new edge preserving Buck's fascia (without dorsal resection) using a suture material *vicryl rapid 5/0* and *monocryl 5/0* in labia and *vicryl rapid 5/0* in clitoral frenulum as shown in Fig. 13.1 [15].

Demonstrating that preoperative sensitivity and at 6 and 12 months postoperatively, there were no changes in hypersensitivity or loss of sensitivity. Labia minora sensitivity could be increased from 2 weeks to 3 months postoperatively, but in a transitory way. No sexual changes were described but an increase of 44.1% in the number of sexual intercourse ($P = 0.011$) due to decreased embarrassment and increased confidence in genital appearance suggesting that the procedure has positive psychological effects [15].

Ethical aspects   This refers mainly to social pressure and autonomy, as there may be a conflict when changing the genital appearance and altering the body to find a desired image. It has been found that, if such motivation is not personal, but is encouraged by third parties or conditioning, it may affect postoperative satisfaction in the long term when the conditioning is released or contact with the third party that encourages the procedure is lost [14]. For this reason, it is important when assessing the patient's motivation that it is genuine and a personal decision.

Symmetry   Up to 57.1% of women may consider that the postoperative appearance does not fully meet their expectations, and this is due to the feeling that their genital appearance is still not "perfect," since prior to surgery they expected to see completely symmetrical labia minora with no protruding labial tissue or completely

Fig. 13.1 Labiaplasty pre- and post-labiaplasty marking. A preoperative and postoperative sensitivity evaluation was performed at 2 weeks, 3, 6, and 12 months at points A, B, C, D, and E using Semmes-Weinstein monofilaments as shown in Fig. 13.2 [15]

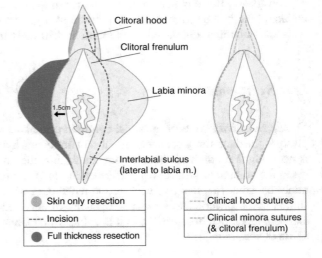

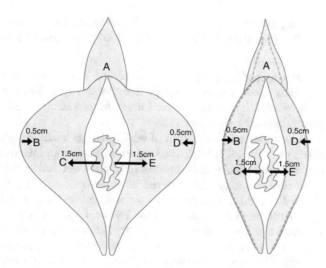

Fig. 13.2 Sensitivity points. One on the clitoral hood and four on the labia minora, 2 stitches 0.5 cm from the edge of the labia minora medially and two stitches 1.5 cm from the hymen towards the labia minora operated on. (Taken from Placik OJ, Arkins JP. A Prospective Evaluation of Female External Genitalia Sensitivity to Pressure following Labia Minora Reduction and Clitoral Hood Reduction. *Plast Reconstr Surg.* 2015;136(4):442e–52e. https://doi.org/10.1097/PRS.0000000000001573)

absent labia minora, and because of this they are a little less satisfied with the results. Even so, in the same publications that indicate this percentage, they state that the patients did not plan to undergo a second procedure and ended up satisfied with an acceptance of improvement but still slightly "imperfect" labia [16].

It has been estimated that approximately 50.7% of women report that they have an idea of what female genitalia look like and almost 47.9% are influenced by the media. Most women have an abnormal perception of their genitalia and consider surgery for more than 6 months after making the decision to have the procedure. This percentage in small study populations is usually not reliable, also because of the possibility of inefficient presurgical counseling that does not rule out body dysmorphism and does not adequately explain the objectives, the natural asymmetry of the human body, and the results of the surgery [3].

Satisfaction and psychological sequelae As mentioned above, labia minora reduction labiaplasty is a highly satisfactory surgery from the psychological and sexual point of view with reported overall satisfaction of 87–97%.

Up to 93% reported improvement in self-esteem, 90% reduction in psychological stress, 71% improvement in sex life, and overall satisfaction with 95% improvement in labia minora discomfort during penetration [1].

Psychosexual outcome Psychosexual outcome after labiaplasty has been evaluated with specific measures of body image and sexual function such as GAS and FSFI where clinically significant and reliable; 96% improvement of the scales has been observed 3 months after the procedure and 91.3% improvement at long-term follow-up [12].

Overall sexual satisfaction is higher in multiparous women than in nulliparous women because they notice a greater change after becoming mothers. An increase of up to 35% in arousal has been observed after the procedure due to improved sexual self-perception and self-esteem [1].

In a publication to evaluate the impact of labiaplasty on sexuality, a self-esteem scale (*Rosemberg*) and the FSFI were applied in two groups; an intervention group where women underwent labiaplasty immediately after answering the first questionnaires and a control group that received no intervention during the 6-month follow-up period. No significant differences were found on the self-esteem scale, but there was a significant improvement in the FSFI total score in the domains of pain and satisfaction and concluded that labiaplasty had a positive impact on sexuality in the study population. Almost all of the women who had experienced sexual difficulties but did not have a diagnosis of *female sexual dysfunction* (83.3%) reported a reduction in their anxieties around sexual intercourse after their labial reduction. However, 33.3% mentioned that some of their difficulties with intercourse and relationships were psychological in origin and were not alleviated by labia minora reduction according to previously reported evidence [17].

Pregnancy and Labiaplasty

Labia minora reduction labiaplasty can be performed before or after pregnancy.

Pregnancy and childbirth involve major adaptations of genitals and pelvic floor to allow the required adaptations for delivery with subsequent return to normal progesterone levels, but such recovery is often incomplete; thus, childbirth has been identified as an important risk factor for both prolapse and changes in pelvic floor function [18].

Like other parts of the body, labia minora respond to the physiological hormonal variations of pregnancy and puerperium. The labia minora increase in size as a result of increased blood flow, which causes distension of blood vessels and increased pelvic pressure with further stretching of the labia, being even greater during vaginal delivery.

The most frequently found is that once the body returns to its basal physiological state, the labia minora tend to return to its prepregnancy state; however, in some cases the skin of the labia minora may present some elongation and flaccidity mainly in multiparous women, making evident the "increase" in size of the labia minora with the passage of time. These changes do not contraindicate the performance of labiaplasty before pregnancy, because the lack of regression is infrequent, and there are few reported cases of labia minora hypertrophy as a clinical finding in the postpartum period.

In a logistic regression analysis assessing factors that may have influenced women's complaints about their labia minora, significant associations were found in women who had undergone previous cosmetic surgery ($P = 0.018$) and women who had an individual perception of "altered" labia minora ($P = 0.03$). Previous pregnancy and labia minora width did not show significant influences in the multivariable regression model [19].

Inside the scarce literature found on the relationship of seeking labiaplasty and pregnancy, the perception of hyperpigmentation of labia minora is found in two thirds of women seeking labiaplasty after one or more pregnancies, and 80% of them relate that this change occurred during adolescence (36.4%) or pregnancy (43.9%) according to the two periods of a woman's life with greater increase in hormonal levels [20].

Hamori et al. point out that recognizing the great variety of size, shape, and color of a body part does not mean that it should not be operated on because of possible harm; just as complications of surgical breast reduction can affect lactation, labiaplasty also carries risks and complications.

In one of the reports, it is observed that in nulliparous patients who underwent labiaplasty, three became pregnant after surgery, two of them ended their pregnancy by vaginal delivery, and one of them with episiotomy; in the latter, slow healing was observed that took up to 3 weeks without pathological implications in any of the cases without reporting recurrences or alterations in the labia minora. It is understood that this is not a crucial publication to draw conclusions about the results and should be considered for future research [21].

In a telephone survey of 204 patients, 70 patients had children before labiaplasty, while 33 had children after labiaplasty. The vaginal delivery rate was lower in women who had children before labiaplasty (82.6% vs. 91.8%, $P = 0.015$). The laceration/episiotomy rate for vaginal deliveries was lower in women who delivered before labiaplasty compared to after labiaplasty (3.1% vs. 17.8%, $P < 0.001$). Among women who delivered only after labiaplasty, the reported tear/episiotomy rate was 7/39 vaginal deliveries (17.9%).

This showed more than 90% success rate with vaginal deliveries after labiaplasty. For nulliparous patients contemplating the procedure, the data suggest that the risk of episiotomy or vaginal tearing with vaginal delivery after labiaplasty is comparable or lower than the general population, further supporting the safety of this procedure. For women with previous deliveries, data is even more limited but do not suggest an increased risk in this study population [22].

Conclusions

Labia minora labiaplasty is a highly satisfactory and safe surgery under expert and trained hands; respecting the anatomy and functionality has not been shown to alter the sensitivity or functionality. This makes it different from genital mutilation;

therefore it is emphasized that the great variety in size, shape, and color of a body part that causes discomfort does not mean that it should not be operated due to possible damage.

It can be assumed that the limited follow-up, or those who do not seek formal follow-up, is due to high satisfaction and a low long-term complication rate.

Factors that may increase the possibility of postoperative sequelae (such as age, smoking, etc.) should always be considered and evaluated, individualizing each case and providing appropriate guidance to each patient.

The application of several validated scales and questionnaires for the evaluation of self-image, self-esteem, and attitudes towards the procedure, sexual dysfunction, and body dysmorphic syndrome is highly useful in the election of patients and is also valid for postoperative evaluation.

It is very important to determine whether patients choose to undergo surgery for purely aesthetic or functional reasons or ultimately in the hope of improving sexual satisfaction because there are many psychological, hormonal, and anatomical causes for sexual dysfunction. Awareness should be raised that labiaplasty is not intended to cure sexual dysfunction, although it does improve a person's sex life.

The consent form should address in addition to the presence of and guidance on complications, early and late symptoms supported by preoperative standing photographs in cephalocaudal direction and in lithotomy.

Annex: Validated Questionnaires to Assess Aesthetic and Functional Aspects Before and After Labiaplasty

Annex 1: COPS-L [11]

COPS-L for Women Seeking Labiaplasty

*This questionnaire is about the way you feel about the appearance of your genitalia. The outer lips of your genitalia are called the "labia" Please answer how you feel for **over the past week**.*

Name _____ Date _____

1. How abnormal do you feel your labia is to a sexual partner (if you do **not try to hide your genitalia**) and you do not highlight it to him/her?

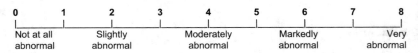

2. To what extent do you feel the appearance of your labia are **currently** ugly, unattractive or 'not right'?

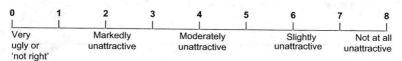

3. To what extent do your labia **currently** cause you distress?

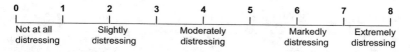

4. To what extent does thinking about the appearance of your labia **currently** preoccupy you? That is, you think about it a lot and it is hard to stop thinking about it?

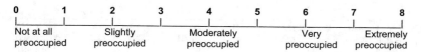

5. If you **have a regular partner**, to what extent do your concerns about your labia **currently** have an effect on your relationship with an existing partner? (e.g. affectionate feelings, number of arguments, enjoying activities together?) **If you do not have a regular partner**, to what extent do your concerns about your labia **currently** have an effect on dating or developing a relationship? (do not include any sexual relationship as this is discussed below).

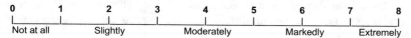

6. If you **have a regular partner**, to what extent do your concerns about your labia **currently** have an effect on an existing sexual relationship? (e.g. enjoyment of sex, frequency of sexual activity, labia getting trapped in your vagina, only having sex in the dark). **If you do not have a regular partner**, to what extent do your concerns about your labia **currently** stop you from developing a sexual relationship?

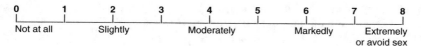

7. To what extent do your concerns about your labia currently interfere with your leisure activities that might involve someone noticing your labia? (e.g., those that might involve public changing rooms or wearing swimsuits)

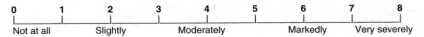

| 0 | 1 | 2 | 3 | 4 | 5 | 6 | 7 | 8 |

Not at all   Slightly   Moderately   Markedly   Very severely

8. How noticeable do you think your labia are in public situations (e.g., in a changing room naked) **if you do not try to deliberately hide your genitalia?**

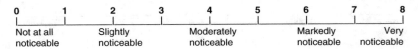

| 0 | 1 | 2 | 3 | 4 | 5 | 6 | 7 | 8 |

Not at all   Slightly   Moderately   Markedly   Very
noticeable   noticeable   noticeable   noticeable   noticeable

9. How do think the appearance of your labia compare to other women of the same age and ethnic group?

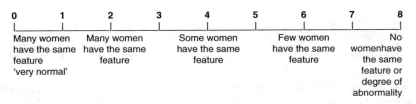

| 0 | 1 | 2 | 3 | 4 | 5 | 6 | 7 | 8 |

Many women   Many women   Some women   Few women   No
have the same   have the same   have the same   have the same   womenhave
feature   feature   feature   feature   the same
'very normal'   feature or
                                                                              degree of
                                                                              abnormality

Annex 2: GAS [11]

Veale, David & Eshkevari, Ertimiss & Ellison, Nell & Cardozo, Linda & Robinson, Dudley & Kavouni, Angelica. (2013). Genital Appearance Satisfaction Scale (Bramwell, 2009).

Below you will find a number of statements that women often make when referring to the genital area, read each one and choose the answer that you feel applies to you. A diagram of the anatomy of the female external genitalia will be provided.

1. I feel that my genitals are normal looking.
   Never—Sometimes—Almost always—Always
2. I feel that my genitals look unattractive.
   Never—Sometimes—Almost always—Always
3. I feel my labia vulvae are too long.
   Never—Sometimes—Almost always—Always
4. I am satisfied with the appearance of my genitals.
   Never—Sometimes—Almost always—Always
5. I experience irritation of my labia when exercising or walking.
   Never—Sometimes—Almost always—Always

6. I feel or have felt conscious of labia size in sexual situations because of the appearance of my genitals.
      Never—Sometimes—Almost always—Always
7. I am embarrassed by the appearance of my genitals, and it limits my enjoyment of sex.
      Never—Sometimes—Almost always—Always
8. I feel discomfort in my genitals when I wear tight clothing.
      Never—Sometimes—Almost always—Always
9. I feel that my genital area is visible through tight clothing.
      Never—Sometimes—Almost always—Always
10. I am concerned about the appearance of my genital area.
      Never—Sometimes—Almost always—Always
11. I feel that my genital area looks asymmetrical or larger on one side.
      Never—Sometimes—Almost always—Always

Annex 3: FSFI: Validated Version in Colombia [13]

Validation P, Sexual F, Index F, Behavior S. 1.2 Validated version in Colombia of The Female Sexual Function Index (FSFI; Rosen et al., 2000). 2017;(61).
   Check only one alternative per question:

1. During the past 4 weeks, how often have you felt sexual desire or interest?

      Always or almost always—5
      Most of the time (more than half the time)—4
      Some of the time (about half the time)—3
      Rarely (less than half the time)—2
      Hardly ever or never—1

2. During the past 4 weeks, how would you rate your level of sexual desire or interest?

      Very high—5
      High—4
      Moderate—3
      Low—2
      Very low or none—1

3. During the past 4 weeks, how often have you felt sexual arousal during sexual activity or intercourse (alone or with a partner)?

      I have not been sexually active—0
      Always or almost always—5
      Most of the time (more than half the time)—4
      Some of the time (about half the time)—3
      Rarely (less than half the time)—2

Hardly ever or never—1

4. During the past 4 weeks, how would you rate your level of sexual arousal during sexual activity or intercourse (alone or with a partner)?

I have not been sexually active—0
Very high—5
High—4
Moderate—3
Low—2
Very low or none—1

5. During the past 4 weeks, how confident were you that you would become sexually aroused during sexual activity or intercourse (alone or with a partner)?

I have not been sexually active—0
Very safe—5
Safe—4
Moderately safe—3
Unsafe—2
Almost nothing or not sure at all—1

6. During the past 4 weeks, how often have you been comfortable with your sexual arousal during sexual activity or intercourse (alone or with a partner)?

I have not been sexually active—0
Always or almost always—5
Most of the time (more than half the time)—4
Some of the time (about half the time)—3
Rarely (less than half the time)—2
Hardly ever or never—1

7. During the past 4 weeks, how often have you been able to stay lubricated ("wet") during sexual activity or intercourse (alone or with a partner)?

I have not been sexually active—0
Always or almost always—5
Most of the time (more than half the time)—4
Some of the time (about half the time)—3
Rarely (less than half the time)—2
Hardly ever or never—1

8. During the past 4 weeks, how difficult has it been for you to lubricate ("get wet") during sexual activity or intercourse (alone or with a partner)?

I have not been sexually active—0
Extremely difficult or impossible—1
Very difficult—2
Hard—3
A bit difficult—4

Nothing difficult—5

9. During the past 4 weeks, how often did you stay lubricated ("wet") until the end of sexual activity or intercourse (alone or with a partner)?

    I have not been sexually active—0
    Always or almost always—5
    Most of the time (more than half of the time)—4
    Some of the time (about half the time)—3
    Rarely (less than half the time)—2
    Hardly ever or never—1

10. During the past 4 weeks, how difficult was it to stay lubricated ("wet") until the end of sexual activity or intercourse (alone or with a partner)?

    I have not been sexually active—0
    Extremely difficult or impossible—1
    Very difficult—2
    Hard—3
    A bit difficult—4
    Nothing difficult—5

11. During the past 4 weeks, when you have had sexual stimulation or intercourse (alone or with a partner), how often did you orgasm ("come")?

    I have not been sexually active—0
    Always or almost always—5
    Most of the time (more than half of the time)—4
    Some of the time (about half the time)—3
    Rarely (less than half the time)—2
    Hardly ever or never—1

12. During the past 4 weeks, when you have had sexual stimulation or intercourse (alone or with a partner), how difficult was it to achieve orgasm ("come")?

    I have not been sexually active—0
    Extremely difficult or impossible—1
    Very difficult—2
    Hard—3
    A bit difficult—4
    Nothing difficult—5

13. During the past 4 weeks, how satisfied have you been with your ability to achieve orgasm ("come") during sexual activity or intercourse (alone or with a partner)?

    I have not been sexually active—0
    Very satisfied—5
    Moderately compliant—4
    Neither satisfied nor dissatisfied—3

Moderately dissatisfied—2
Very unhappy—1

14. During the past 4 weeks, how satisfied have you been with the level of emotional closeness during sexual activity with your partner?

    I have not been sexually active—0
    Very satisfied—5
    Moderately satisfied—4
    Neither satisfied nor dissatisfied—3
    Moderately dissatisfied—2
    Very dissatisfied—1

15. During the past 4 weeks, how satisfied have you been in your sexual relations with your partner?

    Very satisfied—5
    Moderately satisfied—4
    Neither satisfied nor dissatisfied—3
    Moderately dissatisfied—2
    Very dissatisfied—1

16. During the past 4 weeks, how satisfied have you been with your sex life in general?

    Very satisfied—5
    Moderately satisfied—4
    Neither satisfied nor dissatisfied—3
    Moderately dissatisfied—2
    Very dissatisfied—1

17. During the past 4 weeks, how often have you experienced discomfort or pain during vaginal penetration?

    I have not had vaginal penetration—0
    Always or almost always—1
    Most of the time (more than half the time)—2
    Some of the time (about half the time)—3
    Rarely (less than half the time)—4
    Hardly ever or never—5

18. During the past 4 weeks, how often have you felt discomfort or pain after vaginal penetration?

    I have not had vaginal penetration—0
    Always or almost always—1
    Most of the time (more than half the time)—2
    Some of the time (about half the time)—3
    Rarely (less than half the time)—4
    Hardly ever or never—5

19. During the past 4 weeks, how would you rate your level of discomfort or pain during vaginal penetration?

       I have not had vaginal penetration—0
       Very high—1
       High—2
       Moderate—3
       Low—4
       Very low or none—5

FSFI

References

1. Surroca MM, Miranda LS, Ruiz JB. Labiaplasty: a 24-month experience in 58 patients: outcomes and statistical analysis. Ann Plast Surg. 2018;80(4):316–22. https://doi.org/10.1097/SAP.0000000000001395.
2. Sharp G, Tiggemann M, Mattiske J. A retrospective study of the psychological outcomes of labiaplasty. Aesthet Surg J. 2017;37(3):324–31. https://doi.org/10.1093/asj/sjw190.
3. Dogan O, Yassa M. Major motivators and sociodemographic features of women undergoing labiaplasty. Aesthet Surg J. 2019;39(12):NP517–27. https://doi.org/10.1093/asj/sjy321.
4. Oranges CM, Schaefer KM, Kalbermatten DF, Haug M, Schaefer DJ. Why women request labiaplasty. Plast Reconstr Surg. 2017;140(6):829e. https://doi.org/10.1097/PRS.0000000000003871.
5. Hamori CA. Teen labiaplasty: a response to the May 2016 American College of Obstetricians and Gynecologists (ACOG) recommendations on labiaplasty in adolescents. Aesthet Surg J. 2016;36(7):807–9. https://doi.org/10.1093/asj/sjw099.
6. Wood PL. Cosmetic genital surgery in children and adolescents. Best Pract Res Clin Obstet Gynaecol. 2018;48:137–46. https://doi.org/10.1016/j.bpobgyn.2017.08.003.
7. Bucknor A, Chen AD, Egeler S, et al. Labiaplasty: indications and predictors of postoperative sequelae in 451 consecutive cases. Aesthet Surg J. 2018;38(6):644–53. https://doi.org/10.1093/asj/sjx241.
8. Sarwer DB. Body image, cosmetic surgery, and minimally invasive treatments. Body Image. 2019;31:302–8. https://doi.org/10.1016/j.bodyim.2019.01.009.
9. Müllerová J, Weiss P. Plastic surgery in gynaecology: factors affecting women's decision to undergo labiaplasty. Mind the risk of body dysmorphic disorder: a review. J Women Aging. 2020;32(3):241–58. https://doi.org/10.1080/08952841.2018.1529474.
10. De Brito MJA, Nahas FX, Sabino NM. Invited Response on: Body dysmorphic disorder: is there an "ideal" strategy? Aesthet Plast Surg. 2019;43(4):1115–6. https://doi.org/10.1007/s00266-019-01384-8.
11. Veale D, Eshkevari E, Ellison N, Cardozo L, Robinson D, Kavouni A. Validation of genital appearance satisfaction scale and the cosmetic procedure screening scale for women seeking labiaplasty. J Psychosom Obstet Gynaecol. 2013;34(1):46–52. https://doi.org/10.3109/0167482X.2012.756865.
12. Veale D, Naismith I, Eshkevari E, et al. Psychosexual outcome after labiaplasty: a prospective case-comparison study. Int Urogynecol J. 2014;25(6):831–9. https://doi.org/10.1007/s00192-013-2297-2.

13. Vallejo-Medina P, Pérez-Durán C, Saavedra-Roa A. Translation, adaptation, and preliminary validation of the female sexual function index into spanish (Colombia). Arch Sex Behav. 2018;47(3):797–810.
14. Özer M, Mortimore I, Jansma EP, Mullender MG. Labiaplasty: motivation, techniques, and ethics. Nat Rev Urol. 2018;15(3):175–89. https://doi.org/10.1038/nrurol.2018.1.
15. Placik OJ, Arkins JP. A prospective evaluation of female external genitalia sensitivity to pressure following labia minora reduction and clitoral hood reduction. Plast Reconstr Surg. 2015;136(4):442e–52e. https://doi.org/10.1097/PRS.0000000000001573.
16. Sharp G, Mattiske J, Vale KI. Motivations, expectations, and experiences of labiaplasty: a qualitative study. Aesthet Surg J. 2016;36(8):920–8. https://doi.org/10.1093/asj/sjw014.
17. Turini T, Weck Roxo AC, Serra-Guimarães F, et al. The impact of labiaplasty on sexuality. Plast Reconstr Surg. 2018;141(1):87–92. https://doi.org/10.1097/PRS.0000000000003921.
18. Goodman MP. Female genital cosmetic and plastic surgery: a review. J Sex Med. 2011;8(6):1813–25. https://doi.org/10.1111/j.1743-6109.2011.02254.x.
19. Widschwendter A, Riedl D, Freidhager K, et al. Perception of labial size and objective measurements-is there a correlation? A cross-sectional study in a cohort not seeking labiaplasty. J Sex Med. 2020;17(3):461–9. https://doi.org/10.1016/j.jsxm.2019.11.272.
20. Miklos JR, Moore RD. Postoperative cosmetic expectations for patients considering labiaplasty surgery: our experience with 550 patients. Surg Technol Int. 2011;21:170–4.
21. Hamori CA. Aesthetic surgery of the female genitalia: labiaplasty and beyond. Plast Reconstr Surg. 2014;134:661–73.
22. Kearney AM, Turin SY, Placik OJ, Wattanasupachoke L. Incidence of obstetric lacerations and episiotomy following labiaplasty. Aesthet Surg J. 2020;2020:sjaa027. https://doi.org/10.1093/asj/sjaa027.

Chapter 14
Clinical Sexology and Cosmetic Gynecology: An Integral Work for the Benefit of the Patients

Ezequiel López Peralta

A woman worried about the appearance of her vulva, for example, the color, the size, or shape of her labia minora or a redundant clitoral hood, is affected by her self-image. She does not feel comfortable with these features of her body, develops complexes about them, does not fully enjoy her sexuality, or even inhibits certain types of erotic behaviors and games because of embarrassment. Receptive oral sex is a clear example of this.

This negative self-perception affects, logically, her self-esteem. The woman feels devaluated, compares herself with other women, placing her in a position of inferiority, and also attributes that her partner has the same negative perception (which, by the way, does not always correspond to the reality of the sexual partner).

Considering that sexual function has a very important mental component, it is sensible to deduce that these complexes with the body and low self-esteem do not help the performance to be as expected by the woman herself and her partner. Negative thoughts, the so-called *bystander role*, and the aforementioned limitations can affect desire, arousal, orgasm, and all of the above [1, 2].

But let's also remember that the specialty of cosmetic gynecology is also related to functional gynecology, and some interventions are aimed to improve sexual function and pleasure of women. The aging process and natural childbirth, to mention the two most common factors, weakening pelvic floor muscles and vaginal walls, affect their ability to contract and relax. This particularly impacts arousal phase, characterized by vaginal lubrication and dilation, diminishing pleasure and indirectly affecting orgasmic function and desire.

For both ICD 10 (International Classification of Diseases of the World Health Organization) and DSM V (Diagnostic and Statistical Manual of Mental Disorders of the American Psychiatric Association), sexual dysfunction is an alteration in one

E. L. Peralta (✉)
Private Practice, Bogotá, Colombia
e-mail: ezequiel@citaconezequiel.com; https://www.citaconezequiel.com

© The Author(s), under exclusive license to Springer Nature Switzerland AG 2023
P. Gonzalez-Isaza, R. Sánchez-Borrego (eds.), *Topographic Labiaplasty*, https://doi.org/10.1007/978-3-031-15048-7_14

or more phases of the human sexual response. We must establish whether it is primary or secondary, situational or general, of gradual or abrupt onset, its severity (mild to severe), and its etiology (organic, psychological, or mixed).

The study by Laumann, Park, and Rosen on the prevalence of sexual dysfunction in the United States shows that it is higher in women (43%, being more frequent after the age of 45) than in men (31%). On the other hand, the prevalence of female sexual dysfunction between the ages of 40 and 60 ranges from 51% to 66%.

It should be noted that for the most recent version of the Diagnostic and Statistical Manual of Mental Disorders, the DSM V, hypoactive sexual desire, and sexual arousal disorder in women were integrated into the same diagnostic category. It is *sexual and interest arousal disorder (SIAD)*, which includes the following diagnostic criteria:

1. Absent or reduced interest in sexual activity.
2. Absent or reduced sexual/erotic thoughts and fantasies.
3. Lack of initiation of sexual activity and lack of receptivity to the partner's attempts to initiate sexual activity.
4. Absent or reduced sexual arousal and/or pleasure during sexual activity (in all or almost all sexual encounters).
5. Desire is rarely or never triggered by an internal or external erotic stimulus (written, verbal, visual).
6. Absent or reduced genital and/or non-genital sensations during sexual activity (in all or almost all sexual encounters).

These changes are closely related to the good reception in the sexological scientific community of Rosemary Basson's circular model of the female sexual response cycle. According to this author, the sexual desire of approximately half of the women in her sample is not spontaneous but responsive. The mentioned process begins with a space of emotional intimacy, in which an effective sexual stimulus is produced inside an adequate context, from there the physical and subjective arousal, and finally the sexual desire arises.

Finally, I want to refer to the concept of sexual satisfaction. According to Byers et al. [3, 4], it is *an affective response that arises from the evaluation of the positive and negative aspects associated with one's sexual relations.* This evaluation is related to sexual practices, emotional aspects of the couple's relationship, knowledge, attitudes, and values towards sexuality, psychophysical health and vitality, and environmental barriers. Without going into detail on these points, I think it is reasonable to suggest that the limitations that women may have in their erotic encounters as a result of their negative self-perception, sexual satisfaction would be affected and would not reach its maximum expression.

Sexual dissatisfaction is often associated with the wear and tear of the bond itself, unresolved conflicts, accidental situations they have experienced, and their own structural crises. Sexual monotony, understood as the repetition of erotic scripts that have become stereotyped over time, is the most common difficulty and the one that couples feel most disoriented about, as they often think that this problem has no solution. Sexual dyschronaxias or dysrhythmias, that is to say the notable difference in the levels of sexual desire of the couple, generate discussions, misinterpretations, arguments, and conflicts. Sexual communication is not always effective and assertive, and its unresolved disturbances are also a source of sexual problems and disorders, both as a cause and as an effect. We also know that simultaneous relationships, parallel to the stable relationship, are not uncommon and are more probable as the years go by and in situations of marital and sexual dissatisfaction.

At this point, I think it is important to underline that cosmetic gynecology is a specialty that generally involves minimally invasive interventions, so it is legitimate for women to benefit from them in order to adjust their body to their expectations. Thus, their self-perception will be more positive, and possibly other aspects mentioned above will be modified. But of course, for that to happen, some conditions must be met [5]:

- The intervention is under the hands of professionals with the necessary theoretical and technical knowledge, experience, and equipment.
- The patient has reasonable expectations and does not have a diagnosis of body dysmorphic disorder. For this, a psychological evaluation is crucial when there are suspicions of this condition [6].
- Evaluate the woman's sexual function and satisfaction, also involving her partner, before and after the intervention. At this point, ideally, an assessment should be made by a specialist in clinical sexology, who will conduct a focused interview and apply psychometric diagnostic tools such as the Female Sexual Function Index (FSFI, [7–9]) or one of the sexual satisfaction inventories.
- Interventions from clinical sexology as a complement to cosmetic-gynecology intervention. Considering that sexologists generally work with a focused therapy model, we establish together which areas of intervention would be increasing desire, controlling anxiety, facilitating the arousal or orgasm response, promoting erotic enrichment, and training erotic creativity or assertive erotic communication.

In order to expose the model of work in clinical sexology, I will begin by referring to the sexological interview, and then I will present some interventions that fit the objective of reversing sexual dysfunctions and develop erotic skills.

The sexological interview

The sexological consultation has certain particularities that require the development of therapeutic relationship skills among practitioners. Additionally, we need more time than is usually provided in the typical consultation in gynecology or medicine due to the complexity of the patient, the problem, and situation.

One of the outstanding characteristics of our patients is the presence of emotions that do not favor the solution at all, insofar as they are at least partially—causes that produce and maintain the problem that motivates the consultation: shame, anguish, and feelings of guilt—part of a culture that represses the exercise of sexual function, especially when it comes to female pleasure. The same situation of meeting with the professional is difficult to face, and the patient's prejudices are reflected in questions such as "what will he ask me?," "will he think I am a very sick woman?," "will I have to tell things I don't want to?," and "at my age, shouldn't I consult about my sexual health?" Negative emotions about sexuality and the specialized consultation itself are based on false beliefs that are sometimes deeply rooted in the social imaginary, for example:

- The woman's enjoyment is not so important compared to that of the man.
- When we experience sexual problems, it is because our body is already telling us that our sex life is over.
- Sexual problems resolve spontaneously, over time.
- Sexual problems are exclusively psychological and emotional.
- Sexological consultation is only for serious cases, not for sexual orientation and counseling.

These arguments do not resist any analysis, but we cannot deny that inside our culture there are still beliefs that hinder the path to a full sexual life, and therefore we need to work with our patients with a psychoeducational approach.

An additional issue that patients find is that it is not always easy for them to locate a sexology specialist. They are afraid to go inside an institute or professional who is not properly trained and accredited. Therefore, to the extent that the gynecological consultation is not enough to solve sexual demands from the patient, it is essential that we have trusted professionals to whom we can refer.

In psychotherapy, we know that *rapport* or therapeutic alliance is key to the achievement of the planned objectives. Let's look at some basic therapeutic skills to implement in the sexological interview.

Show compassion for the patient's suffering It is not enough for us to know that this is a different consultation for the patient; we also have to let her know, show her that it is very clear to us that it is not easy to be in her place, reinforce her courage to overcome prejudices and, verbally express to her that it is clear to us how difficult it is to deal with a sexual problem.

Unconditional acceptance It is to explicitly express that we are prepared to listen to everything the patient has to tell us and that therefore should not be afraid since our concept of her will not change. In contrast, we value her sincerity as a positive characteristic to help her.

Establishing an explicit alliance Psychotherapy and sex therapy as a focused treatment require a manifest agreement—that some therapists even make in writing—in which each one commits to form a partnership. Within this scheme, the parties have a function, certain tasks, and also a timeline to reach the partial and final goals.

Handle with warmth and cordiality Let's think of a patient whom have already pointed out an important burden of anguish and many taboos to overcome. The treatment should be close, warm, and with an appropriate body language for the situation: sustained look, posture of tranquility and security, supportive smile, and perhaps some physical contact such as a pat on the back or a slight squeeze on the shoulders. However, be especially careful with physical contact with patients who have been sexually abused, and with those who are particularly structured and formal, who may misinterpret the situation.

Demonstrate knowledge, confidence, and expertise Handling statistical data—which may include your own casuistry—about the problem that is the reason for the consultation, explaining the diagnostic tests to be performed, asking questions that evaluate aspects that the patient herself never thought about, and going into the different types of treatments that exist—including those that we do not handle ourselves—is a demonstration of professionalism and expertise.

Keep the focus of the interview We can allocate more or less time to the interview, but it is always limited. That is why we must keep the focus of the intervention and do not let the patient manage the therapeutic timeframe. Some patients show a phobic characteristic and avoid touching on certain contents—addressing them superficially or changing the subject—that we consider important. Others are vague and diffuse in their thinking and do not focus on what is relevant, so we must focus on them. In summary we must always maintain leadership and control of the interview; otherwise we run the risk of losing hierarchy and a good therapeutic approach.

Motivate for change by instilling hope Motivation is a big part of therapeutic success, and that is why we need a professional with a motivating personality, especially considering the high level of hopelessness of the patient with sexual dysfunction—even more so when it is chronic or previous failed treatments. How do we motivate? With a very positive attitude, explaining how we are going to achieve the objectives, showing studies that prove the effectiveness of sex therapy, rewarding the patient with a congratulation when she follows assignments and progresses, and also putting the solution in her hands, since in fact the solution depends deeply on her compromise and efforts.

Avoid letting one's own personal conflicts and situations affect the therapeutic process Particular issues, particular situations, or certain personality types of the patient may touch on limitations that—like any person—we have in relation to sexuality. If this affects the therapeutic process, it is ethically correct to refer the patient to another professional.

The anamnesis is composed, primarily, about the collection of elementary data as part of the design of the clinical history and, on the other hand, of questions that are key in the sexological interview. We are going to start with basic questions applicable to different reasons for consultation, that will allow us to establish—among other things—the severity of the dysfunction, its evolution, the differential diagnosis, and an approach to its etiology.

The sexual problem It is the reason for consultation or "main complaint" expressed by the patient. In some cases, it is the focus of the therapeutic intervention, while in others we find other underlying problems.

- How would you describe your problem?
- When did the problem start?
- Did the problem start abruptly or gradually?
- Does the problem occur in all circumstances or randomly?

- Under what circumstances does the problem not occur? Describe them.
- What have you tried to do about it?
- What do you think are the causes of your problem?
- How do you feel at the moment the problem occurs?

Intervention in Clinical Sexology

In relation to the intervention in clinical sexology, in the MDS III (Diagnostic Manual in Sexology), Fernando Bianco conceptualizes sexology as *the branch of scientific knowledge that studies sex and sexual function and as an operative concept the branch of scientific knowledge that studies sex, its development process, and alterations* (Tables 14.1 and 14.2). This concept arises from the concept of scientific societies such as FLASSES (Latin American Federation of Sexology and Sex Education Societies), AISM (International Academy of Medical Sexology), and WASM (World Association of Sexual Medicine).

In the following charts, I point out some general and specific techniques in clinical sexology that can be used both for the treatment of different sexual dysfunctions and for the erotic enrichment of the woman and her partner, increasing their sexual satisfaction. In each case I will give a general description, specific objectives, and recommendations (Tables 14.3, 14.4, 14.5, 14.6, 14.7, 14.8, 14.9, 14.10, 14.11, and 14.12).

Psychoeducation

Table 14.1 Psychoeducation

Description	We provide information to the patient related to her specific complaint and other sexual aspects that might be relevant. We have a support from medical references, web sites, tv programs, and education videos
Objectives	To provide scientific information about sexuality, pointing out the reasons for consultation Reduce the negative impact of distorted information about sexual response and satisfaction
Recommendations	Considering that during a sexological consultation misconceptions distorted beliefs and tabus can be found is important to use this kind of tools

Anxiety Management

Table 14.2 Anxiety management

Description	Among sexual dysfunctions there is always some degree of anxiety; hence relaxation is a crucial technical tool. In general Jacobson techniques that use soft breath movements, relaxing thoughts, and movements of contraction-relaxation of muscular groups are effective tools
Objectives	To learn how to relax in specific situations like sexual intercourse Control anxiety by regulating negative thoughts Improve body sensations
Recommendations	It is recommendable to perform relaxation techniques inside our offices, to be aware that the patient comprehends the methodology

Table 14.3 Kegel exercises

Description	They consist of voluntarily contract the pelvic muscles, alternating contraction and relaxation times. There are different exercise protocols, but initially we can work as follows: the patient performs three daily sessions of ten contractions each, during the first week. Then alternate sessions of slow movements with contractions of 5–10 s, with sessions of fast movements, and with contractions of 2 s. The number of contractions per session will increase week by week, until at least they can be triplicated
Objectives	Tonification of pelvic floor muscles Differentiate between contraction and of pelvic muscles Improve genital sensations Improve pleasure during an orgasm
Recommendations	We can start by performing the exercise with small weights and metal balls to be sure that the patients perform the protocol adequately

Table 14.4 Sexual fantasy inventory

Description	The excercise is related to elaborating an exhaustive list of erotic thoughts (fantasies) also a detailed list of all therefore plays and erotic thoughts (fantasies) that produce high degree of pleasure. Once this list of fantasies is completed, must be organized hierarchically according to the sexual arouse by thinking of it. Afterwards results are used according to the objective of the intervention (e.g., to improve sexual desire)
Objectives	To stimulate positive erotic thoughts To be aware of different sexual fantasies To learn how to prioritize sexual fantasies according to the level of sexual arousal they generate
Recommendations	It is not necessary that couples discuss their sexual fantasies to the sexual therapist; the most important thing is to identify and use them accordingly

Table 14.5 Training with erotic images

Description	Point images are selected as the most exciting inside the hierarchy of sexual fantasies inventory. Afterwards we indicate that in a status of relaxation bring them to mind for 10 min twice a day
Objectives	Use of erotic images as a mechanism to stimulate sexual motivation and deactivate negative thoughts related to sexual dysfunctions To enhance physical sensations To overcome sexual inhibitions
Recommendations	It is quite interesting as positive reinforcer to combine the exercise with physical auto-stimulation including genitals

Table 14.6 Genital self-exploration

Description	Consist of performing a complete and detailed self-exploration of genitals step by step. It is necessary to take time and have privacy. A lubricant can be used to aid the process. All general genital anatomy must be identified and stimulated afterwards to identify the most sensitive areas and also the most effective techniques
Objectives	To improve the recording of genital sensations To know different ways to stimulate To be prepared for different stages of the treatment
Recommendations	In patients with taboos related to self-stimulation or even phobia to physical contact, it's convenient to require permission and indicate a relaxation technique previously to the exercise

Table 14.7 Prohibition of intercourse

Description	We ask the couple for a limited specified time (example 2 weeks) to avoid sexual intimacy with penetration. The frame of time can be extended if it's necessary
Objectives	To reduce anxiety and conflicts generated by a sexual contact Enhance noncoital techniques To deactivate a dysfunctional learning
Recommendations	The couple is allowed to have other types of sexual contact including orgasm. When this indication is unfulfilled and had a sexual intercourse, even if it was successful, we encourage the couple again to avoid penetrative sexual contact

Table 14.8 Sensory targeting sensual massage

Description	Is a task to be performed by the couple, it is related to an erotic massage by turns, of not less than 30 min. Oils and reams can be used for the body, for a more pleasurable contact
Objectives	Degenitalize sexuality To relax in couple To improve anxiety and requirements for sexual performance Learn to focus in self sensations Start a sexual contact con with soft stimuli and prolonged times with no rush
Recommendations	During the exercise contact with genitals or breasts, must be, it is also desirable to avoid sexual intercourse afterwards

Table 14.9 Sensory targeting mutual sexual exploration

Description	Authors proposal is to investigate by turns genitals of the couple. A sensual massage can be performed first, allowing enough time for each other. It is recommendable to use cream or oil for the body; in this way the hands will move easier, and the contact is more enjoyable. Like in the sensual massage, caresses are performed by with separated roles (the one who gives and the one who receives), this facilitates the couple in each role
Objectives	To improve the recording of genital sensations To learn how to stimulate genitals without having an orgasm as an objective To know different sexual preferences of the couple, related to sexual stimulation
Recommendations	Good verbal communication is important during the exercise pointing out which areas produce more or less pleasure

Table 14.10 Modification of erotic scripts

Description	We understand as an *erotic script* the pattern of sexual interactions of the couple. Some scripts are more rigid, and others more flexible and creative. The couple identifies conducts and guidelines of interaction inside their erotic script that needs to be modified
Objectives	To recognize mechanical aspects and unsatisfactory aspects of the sexual script To introduce variations inside the stages of the sexual encounter, pre-coital foreplay, intercourse, and postcoital attitudes
Recommendations	To guide the couple with questions, considering that not all of them point out in detail their sexual script

Table 14.11 Evaluation of sexual activators and inhibitors

Description	A detailed analysis of different erotic stimuli that inhibit or enhance sexual desire is performed. We do not only include what is going on inside the sexual scene specifically, but the daily context inside the erotic relationship. In this way we can evaluate if inside it there are few activators and more inhibitors
Objectives	To recognize stimuli related to activation or inhibition of sexual desire To suggest modifications of the sexual script, increasing activators and reducing inhibitors of sexual desire
Recommendations	It is convenient to perform it individually, so the partner cannot interfere inside the interview

Table 14.12 Sexual aids

Description	Technological advances allow us to have huge possibilities about sexual aids that can be used among all the alternatives we have; as sexual therapist we recommend specifically vibrators for women with anorgasmia. These dispositives are particularly interesting when it comes to facilitate. In women that need a level of stimulation that cannot be achieved by sexual intercourse, genital stimulation, or even oral sex in these cases, small vibrators with different speeds are recommended; in this way the patient can explore the desired speed to have an adequate stimulation
Objectives	To increase the intensity of genital stimulation in order to be closer to the orgasmic threshold
Recommendations	The couple establishes an agreement regarding the sexual aid or the method to be used, always guided by their sexual therapist who must have information regarding different options of sexual toys. It is better that in the first stage to perform the sexual exploration in privacy and afterwards with her couple

Conclusions

Sex therapy is often a difficult challenge: to act in a simplified way in a clinically complex scenario. Because not only the patient and her circumstances require a multiaxial analysis, but the same sexological intervention has so many variants and models that we must choose the most appropriate one. As a university professor once said, "the technique should be adapted to the patient, not the patient to the technique." We need to broaden our view to assess the different diagnostic levels, match with different specialties, choose the focus of intervention, work with persistence, make partial evaluations that sometimes modify the diagnosis and the lines of intervention, and also work the therapeutic relationship with the patient as a tool for changes. In addition, we must not forget the partner who is part of the problem and the solution, so it is advisable to include him/her in the interviews and in the design of the treatment plan.

We hope that this chapter has contributed to stimulate a more integral view of the processes of intervention in cosmetic and functional gynecology, promoting a collaborative work among different specialties.

References

1. Alarcón R. Psychology of happiness. Lima: Universitaria; 2009.
2. Alvarez-Gayou JL. Integral sex therapy. Mexico: Manual Moderno; 2002.
3. Bianco F, et al. Manual de Técnicas Sexuales. Caracas: CIPV; 2010.
4. Byers ES, Demmons S, Lawrence K. Sexual satisfaction within dating relationships: a test of the interpersonal exchange model of sexual satisfaction. J Soc Pers Relat. 1998;15:257–67.
5. Cabello Santamaría F. Medical manual of sexual therapy. Madrid: Psimática; 2002.

6. Hooper A. Sex toys. New York: Dorling Kindersley; 2003.
7. Nappi RE, Lachowsky M. Menopause and sexuality: prevalence of symptoms and impact on quality of life. Maturitas. 2009;63(2):138–41.
8. Othmer E, Othmer S. DSM-IV. The clinical interview. Barcelona: Masson; 1996.
9. Rosen R, Brown C, Heiman J, Leiblum S, Meston C, Shabsigh R, Ferguson D, D'Agostino R. The Female Sexual Function Index (FSFI): a multidimensional self-report instrument for the assessment of female sexual function. J Sex Marital Ther. 2000;26:191–208.

Further Reading

1. American Psychiatric Association. Diagnostic and statistical manual of mental disorders. 4th ed. Washington, DC: American Psychiatric Association; 1994.
2. American Psychiatric Association. DSM-5: the future of psychiatric diagnosis. 2012. www.dsm5.org.
3. Arrington R, Cofrancesco J, Wu AW. Questionnaires to measure sexual quality of life. Qual Life Res. 2004;13:1643–58.
4. Basson R, Berman J, Burnett A, Derogatis L, Ferguson D, Fourcroy J, et al. Report of the International Consensus Development Conference on Female Sexual Dysfunction: definitions and classifications. J Urol. 2000;163:888–93.
5. Basson M, et al. ISSM (International Society of Sexual Medicine). Recommendation for womens sexual dysfunction. 2012. http://www.issm.info/images/book/Committee%2027/#/1/.
6. Beck A. Love is not enough. Barcelona: Paidós; 1990.
7. Bianco F, et al. Diagnostic manual in sexology. 3rd ed. Caracas: CIPV; 2012.
8. Conrad S, Milburn M. Sexual intelligence. Barcelona: Planeta Divulgación; 2002.
9. Elías-Calles L, Machado Porro M (2006). Some considerations about PADAM syndrome. Cuban J Endocrinol. 17(2).
10. Gaja R. Vivir en pareja. Barcelona: De Bolsillo; 2005.
11. Gindín L. La nueva sexualidad de la mujer. Buenos Aires: Norma; 2004.
12. Kaplan H. The sexual desire disorders: dysfunctional regulation of sexual motivation. New York: Brunner/Mazel; 1995.
13. Hooper A. Sexual fantasies. Barcelona: Robinbook; 2003.
14. Johnson V, Masters W. Human sexual response. Buenos Aires: Intermedica; 1981.
15. Laumann EO, Paik A, Rosen RC. Sexual dysfunction in the United States. Prevalence and predictors. JAMA. 1999;281:537–44.
16. López Peralta E. El erotismo infinito. Bogotá: Grijalbo; 2012.
17. López Peralta E. El placer de seducir. Bogotá: Grijalbo; 2014.
18. López Peralta E. Confessions of a Bessologist. Bogotá: Grijalbo; 2016.
19. López Peralta E. Erotic chronicles. Bogotá: Sin Fronteras; 2018.
20. López Peralta E. Guía práctica del erotismo infinito. Bogotá: Grijalbo; 2019.
21. Dennerstein L, Alexander JL, Kotz K. The menopause and sexual functioning: a review of the population-based studies. Annu Rev Sex Res. 2003;14(1):64–82. https://doi.org/10.1080/10532528.2003.10559811.

Chapter 15
Labia Majora Labiaplasty with Hyaluronic Acid

Eva Guisantes

Introduction

Hyaluronic Acid

Hyaluronic acid (HA) is a mucopolysaccharide of the glycosaminoglycan family consisting of chains of *N*-acetylglucosamine and glucuronic acid. It was first isolated in 1934 from the vitreous body of cow eyes by the German pharmacist Karl Meyer at Columbia University. Its name is formed from the words hyal (vitreous) and uronic acid.

HA is a highly hydrophilic gelatinous substance, i.e., with a high hygroscopic or water uptake capacity, preserving the aqueous balance of tissues. It is one of the structural elements of the extracellular matrix of connective tissue together with collagen and elastin. It intervenes in the regeneration processes of damaged tissues. It facilitates cell migration in cases of inflammation and has an anti-inflammatory effect by regulating certain cytokines [1]. Since it is a carbohydrate and not a protein, it is a minimally immunogenic compound.

It is widely distributed in the body in skin, mucous membranes, cartilage (especially in hyaline cartilage), tendons, ligaments, bones, joints (especially in synovial fluid since it is a natural lubricant), and in the vitreous humor. Its functions in bones, tendons, and ligaments as cushioning, support, and tension of tissues. HA levels decline with age.

HA meets the characteristics that any injectable filler material must meet, it is biocompatible, minimally antigenic, nontoxic, and long lasting but not permanent, with an adequate cost, and it is also reversible because it is possible to degrade it with hyaluronidase.

E. Guisantes (✉)
Plastic Surgery Department, Hospital de Terrassa, Barcelona, Spain

© The Author(s), under exclusive license to Springer Nature
Switzerland AG 2023
P. Gonzalez-Isaza, R. Sánchez-Borrego (eds.), *Topographic Labiaplasty*,
https://doi.org/10.1007/978-3-031-15048-7_15

147

There are different types and textures of HA, with different rheological properties. The viscoelastic properties of HA will depend on the cross-linking of the free HA chains, the molecular weight of the chains, the concentration, the length of the chains, and the presence or absence of free HA. Cross-linking is the chemical process that transforms free soluble HA into an insoluble viscoelastic gel using a cross-linking agent to give greater stability to the free HA chains. The higher the degree of cross-linking and cohesiveness, the more durable the HA gel is, the more elastic it is (i.e., the greater its capacity to recover its original shape when a force is applied), and the greater its volumizing capacity, but it loses its water retention capacity (hygroscopic capacity). In the case of the treatment of vulvovaginal atrophy, the HA used to treat labia majora atrophy will have different rheological properties than the HA used to treat the vaginal walls and vestibule.

Atrophy of the Labia Majora of the Vulva

The labia majora undergo changes with age that affect their appearance and function. There is an atrophy of the adipose tissue of the labia majora, which leads to a loss of volume of them. The connective tissues also suffer a laxity that causes a loss of elasticity of labia majora and the appearance of wrinkles. It is frequent in the context of the genitourinary syndrome of the menopause [2–8], whether physiological or due to other causes, but it can also be due to childbirth, to certain sporting practices or weight changes. Labia majora have several functions. Mainly they have a mechanical function of shock absorption in sexual intercourse, in sports, also to avoid the sensation of rubbing against clothing or ambulation. They also have a protective function of the vaginal introitus, keeping it closed, thus preventing the vagina from losing its natural moisture and protecting it against infections. Also, an aesthetic function, a smooth and full labia majora is a sign of youth. When the labia majora atrophies, they lose turgor and leave the vaginal introitus exposed, giving an aged appearance to the external female genitalia and functional discomfort such as increased vaginal dryness, dyspareunia, vaginal pH imbalances, recurrent infections, feelings of increased friction, and irritation. Treatment of labia majora atrophy with HA can improve function, aesthetics, and patient confidence, which positively influences a woman's sexual life [9–13]. Filling of the labia majora is also a good complement to labiaplasty surgery in those patients who suffer from hypertrophy of the labia minora and atrophy of the labia majora, thus achieving better results than with labiaplasty alone.

Labia majora augmentation can also be performed with autologous fat grafting, dermal fat grafts, or local flaps; however, HA allows us to make a fast correction in the office, without downtime or the need for a surgical procedure [14–18].

Selection of Hyaluronic Acid for Labia Majora Augmentation

The HA gel of choice for treating labia majora atrophy should have high viscoelasticity, projection capacity, high cross-linking, good strength, cohesiveness, and volumizing capacity. It is therefore a dense gel. It will allow to resist the mechanical load to which the labia majora is subjected and also should have minimal risk of deformation, fragmentation, or migration, with long-lasting properties.

Injection Technique

Anesthesia

Topical anesthesia is usually insufficient for the injection of the labia majora, so local infiltrative anesthesia is recommended to block the labial and perineal nerves. After asepsis, an anterograde longitudinal anesthetic infiltration is performed along the lateral part of the labia majora (close to the groin). Direct anesthetic injection in the labia majora is avoided because it is more painful and because it distorts the volume of it, making it difficult to assess the immediate aesthetic result of the HA injection. To avoid multiple anesthetic punctures, it is useful to use a long needle 70 mm in length and 25 G in diameter, which allows the entire area to be anesthetized longitudinally from a single entry point located in an anterior position (Fig. 15.1). This same point of entry of the anesthetic needle will be the point of entry of the cannula with which the HA is injected. It is not necessary to associate vasoconstrictor to the local anesthetic. Lidocaine at 1% or mepivacaine at 1% or 2% can be used, in a total amount not exceeding 10 mL (5 mL per labia). Shaving is not necessary. An anesthetic pudendal nerve block may also be performed instead of infiltrative local anesthesia.

It is an outpatient treatment Labia majora labia plasty injection technique anatomy that can be performed inside the doctor's office.

Fig. 15.1 Injection of local anesthetic to anesthetize the labia majora

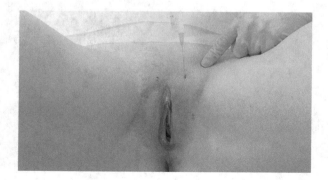

Anatomy of the Labia Majora and Injection Technique

The layers of the labia majora from superficial to deep are the skin, the superficial fascia (intimately attached to the dermis), the subcutaneous adipose tissue that in the labia majora forms an adipose sac, the deep fascia, the bulbospongiosus muscle, and the vestibular bulb (erectile fibroelastic tissue of the labia majora) (Figs. 15.2 and 15.3). Atrophy affects the subcutaneous adipose tissue of the labia majora, and it is in this subcutaneous plane (between the superficial fascia and the adipose sac) that HA gel is deposited (Fig. 15.4). The dermis and superficial fascia resist the passage of the cannula, and this resistance must be overcome to ensure that we are in the subcutaneous plane, where the resistance to the passage of the cannula is lower (Fig. 15.5).

The HA gel indicated for this area must be dense, so it is not advisable to inject it in an intradermal plane due to the risk of palpable nodules. The injection can be performed with either a needle or a cannula. The advantages of the cannula are that it is less traumatic, allows better feeling of the anatomical plane in which we are located, and also is less painful. The cannula to be used must have a sufficient caliber to overcome the resistance of the dermis and superficial fascia and also a sufficient length to be able to inject longitudinally the entire length of labia majora from a single site of injection. The entry point of the cannula may be located at the anterior or posterior aspect of the vulva. A cannula 70–80 mm long and 18 G in diameter is usually used. The cannula should be introduced parallel to the skin to avoid injury to the vestibular bulb during the pressure maneuver required to pass through the

Fig. 15.2 Anatomy of the labia majora

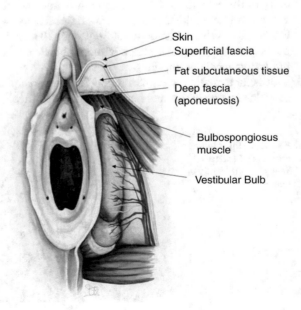

Skin

Superficial fascia

Fat subcutaneous tissue

Deep fascia (aponeurosis)

Bulbospongiosus muscle

Vestibular Bulb

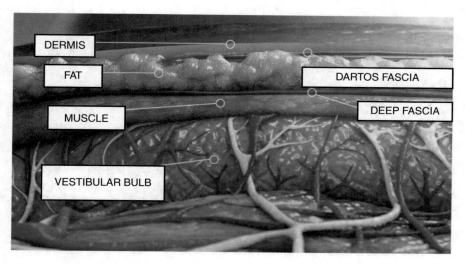

Fig. 15.3 Illustration showing sagittal view of the anatomy of the labia majora

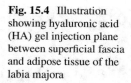

Fig. 15.4 Illustration showing hyaluronic acid (HA) gel injection plane between superficial fascia and adipose tissue of the labia majora

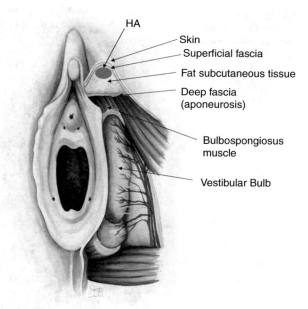

initial resistance of dermis and superficial fascia (Fig. 15.6). The vestibular bulb is a highly vascularized structure and injury to it may result in hematoma formation. Inserting the cannula perpendicular to the skin increases the risk of injury to the bulb. HA injection should not be performed too deep to avoid migration of the product into the ischiorectal fossa, which would waste the product without volumetric

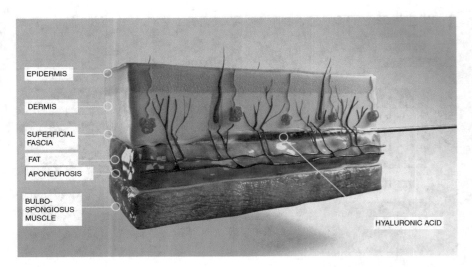

EPIDERMIS

DERMIS

SUPERFICIAL FASCIA

FAT

APONEUROSIS

BULBO-SPONGIOSUS MUSCLE

HYALURONIC ACID

Fig. 15.5 Illustration of sagittal section of the labium majus showing hyaluronic acid gel injection plane between Dartos superficial fascia and adipose tissue

Fig. 15.6 Hyaluronic acid gel injection technique with cannula in the labia majora

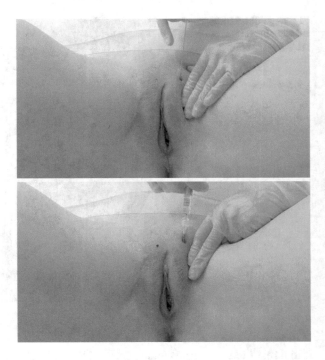

result in the labia majora. HA is injected in a retrograde movement, i.e., HA is injected as the cannula is withdrawn, from distal to proximal with respect to the entry point of the cannula. It is usually necessary to inject 1–2 cc of HA per labia majora. After the injection, the area is gently massaged.

Posttreatment Effects

The volume restoration of the labia majora improves their aesthetic appearance, their mechanical function, and their protective function. The effect lasts between 10 and 12 months. It is advisable to avoid sexual intercourse, saunas, and swimming pools for 1 week. It is not necessary to prescribe antibiotics. Otherwise, the patient can lead a normal life (Figs. 15.7, 15.8, 15.9, and 15.10).

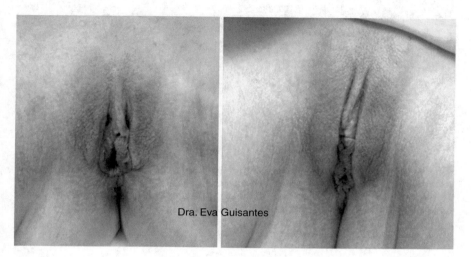

Fig. 15.7 A 41-year-old woman. Injection of HA 1 cc per labia majora. On the left pre-treatment image and on the right posttreatment image

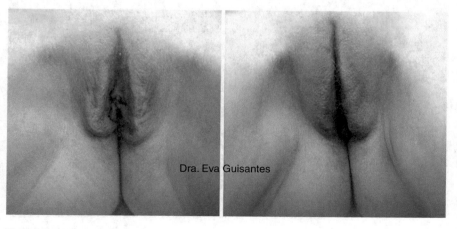

Fig. 15.8 A 58-year-old woman. Injection of HA 2 cc per labia majora. On the left pre-treatment image and on the right posttreatment image

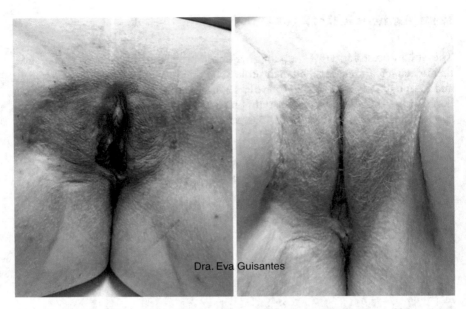

Fig. 15.9 A 42-year-old woman with a history of mastectomy, pharmacological menopause, and breast reconstruction with TMG flap (*transverse musculocutaneous gracilis flap*), who presented right inguinal scar, retraction of the right labia majora, and atrophy of the labia majora. On the left pre-treatment image and on the right posttreatment image

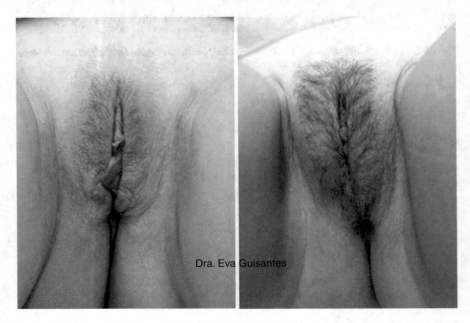

Fig. 15.10 A 55-year-old woman. Injection of HA 1 cc per labia majora. On the left pre-treatment image and on the right posttreatment image

Complications

Complications are rare and are usually related to an inadequate injection technique or choice of product. If they occur, they are usually mild and reversible.

In the case of an injection that is too deep, a hematoma may appear due to a lesion of the vestibular bulb or a migration of the product towards the ischiorectal fossa with the consequent lack of correction of the atrophy of the labia majora. In the case of hematoma, it will be treated as hematomas are usually treated, i.e., local cold, compression, and drainage in case of tension hematoma with skin involvement. The migration of the product has no major consequences for the patient beyond the lack of correction.

In the case of a too superficial intradermal injection with a volumizing gel with the aforementioned characteristics, palpable nodules may appear. Nodules may also appear if an excessive bolus deposit is made at a single injection point. Initially they can be treated with massage. If these nodules persist for more than 6–8 weeks despite massage, they can be treated by injection of hyaluronidase to degrade the gel and thus dissolve the nodules.

Infections are rare and are usually due to a lack of asepsis during the procedure, hence the importance of not touching the cannula with the gauze, gloves, etc. and maintaining basic aseptic measures throughout the process (disinfection, sterile materials, and gloves). Remember that HA gel is sterile, as are the cannula and needle, but not the syringe. Therefore, the needle or cannula must not come into contact with anything except the patient's disinfected skin.

Other mild complications include erythema, edema, pain, or reactivation of genital herpes.

A HA gel with unsuitable viscoelastic properties will not achieve the desired volumizing effect, will degrade too quickly due to increased gel fragmentation, or will migrate.

Intravascular injection into the labium majus is very unlikely, and in general, the use of a cannula is preferable to avoid this complication.

Acknowledgements Thanks to Isdin® and 3D Tech Omega Zeta (http://3dtechomegazeta.com) for providing some of the images used in this chapter. Illustrations: Marina Guisantes.

References

1. Kazezian Z, et al. Injectable hyaluronic acid down-regulates interferon signaling molecules, IGFBP3 and IFIT3 in the bovine intervertebral disc. Acta Biomater. 2017;1(52):118–29.
2. Portman DJ, Gass MLS, Vulvovaginal Atrophy Terminology Consensus Conference Panel. Genitourinary syndrome of menopause: new terminology for vulvo-vaginal atrophy from the International Society for the Study of Women's Sexual Health and The North American Menopause Society. Menopause. 2014;21(10):1063–8.
3. Dennerstein L, et al. A prospective population-based study of menopausal symptoms. Obstet Gynecol. 2000;96(3):351–8.

4. Stenberg A, et al. Prevalence of genitourinary and other climacteric symptoms in 61-year-old women. Maturitas. 1996;24(1–2):31–6.
5. Chim H, et al. The prevalence of menopausal symptoms in a community in Singapore. Maturitas. 2002;41(4):275–82.
6. Faubion SS, et al. Genitourinary syndrome of menopause: management strategies for the clinician. Mayo Clin Proc. 2017;92(12):1842–9.
7. Macbride MB, et al. Vulvovaginal atrophy. Mayo Clin Proc. 2010;85:87–94.
8. Levine KB, et al. Vulvovaginal atrophy is strongly associated with female sexual dysfunction among sexually active postmenopausal women. Menopause. 2008;15:661–6.
9. Fasola E, Gazzola R. Labia majora augmentation with hyaluronic acid filler: technique and results. Aesthet Surg J. 2016;36(10):1155–63.
10. Hexsel D, Dal'Forno T, Caspary P, Hexsel CL. Soft-tissue augmentation with hyaluronic acid filler for labia majora and mons pubis. Dermatol Surg. 2016;42(7):911–4.
11. Jabbour S, et al. Labia majora augmentation: a systematic review of the literature. Aesthet Surg J. 2017;37(10):1157–64.
12. Zerbinati N, et al. A new hyaluronic acid polymer in the augmentation and restoration of labia majora. J Biol Regul Homeost Agents. 2017;31(2):153–61.
13. Fasola E, Anglana F, Basile S, Bernabei G, Cavallini M. A case of labia majora augmentation with hyaluronic acid implant. J Plast Dermatol. 2010;6:215–8.
14. Vogt PM, Herold C, Rennekampff HO. Autologous fat transplantation for labia majora reconstruction. Aesthet Plast Surg. 2011;35:913–5.
15. Hersant B, et al. Labia majora augmentation combined with minimal labia minora resection: a safe and global approach to the external female genitalia. Ann Plast Surg. 2018;80(4):323–7.
16. Karabağlı Y, et al. Labia majora augmentation with de-epithelialized labial rim (minora) flaps as an auxiliary procedure for labia minora reduction. Aesthet Plast Surg. 2015;39(3):289–93.
17. Wilkie G, Bartz D. Vaginal rejuvenation: a review of female genital cosmetic surgery. Obstet Gynecol Surv. 2018;73(5):287–92.
18. Salgado CJ, Tang JC, Desrosiers AE. Use of dermal fat graft for augmentation of the labia majora. J Plast Reconstr Aesthet Surg. 2012;65(2):267–70.

Chapter 16
Clitoropexy-Clitoroplasty

Ricardo L. Kruse

Introduction

Clitoromegaly is a relatively rare condition; nevertheless, its occurrence has been increasing during the last few years due to exogenous hormonal intake among healthy subjects. Although objective measurements defining clitoromegaly vary in literature, its clinical aspect is quite evident to experienced practitioners. There are many causes for clitoromegaly, being the congenital conditions the most common ones, such as classic congenital adrenal hyperplasia. Treatment for clitoromegaly is mainly surgical, yet clitoroplasty is rarely performed in adults. The aim of this chapter is to describe a personal technique to treat adult patients with clinical clitoromegaly, clitoral hypersensitivity due to clitoral overexposure, or clitoral ptosis with safety, adequate aesthetic, and sexually functional results.

Historical Data and Anatomical Considerations

Clitoral hypertrophy is a relative rare condition with sparse data in the literature [1]. The concept of clitoromegaly in literature varies. Oyama defined it as a clitoral area greater than 35–45 mm^2 [2]. According to Tagatz, clitoromegaly is defined as enlarged clitoral size with clitoral glans length more than 10 mm or clitoral index more than 35 mm^2 [3]. The most common cause of clitoromegaly described in literature is classic congenital adrenal hyperplasia. Acquired clitoral enlargement is relatively rare in adult females and occurs under a variety of circumstances [4]. The

R. L. Kruse (✉)
RK—Cirurgia Plástica, Fortaleza, Ceará, Brazil
e-mail: contato@ricardokruse.com.br

© The Author(s), under exclusive license to Springer Nature
Switzerland AG 2023
P. Gonzalez-Isaza, R. Sánchez-Borrego (eds.), *Topographic Labiaplasty*,
https://doi.org/10.1007/978-3-031-15048-7_16

etiologies of acquired clitoromegaly can be categorized as hormonal, nonhormonal, pseudoclitoromegaly, and idiopathic clitoromegaly [5]. In the hormonal causes, an androgen excess is the main contributing factor of the clitoral enlargement. Three groups should be distinguished within this group: endocrinopathies, androgen-producing tumors [6], or exogenous synthetic hormone administrations. The most important endocrinopathies are nonpolycystic ovarian hypertestosteronism and polycystic ovarian syndrome (PCOS) [6]. More recently, there has been a significant increase in clinical clitoromegaly, mostly among gym-goers, bodybuilders, and bioidentical hormone replacement therapy patients, due to synthetic androgen administration (anabolic steroids and androgen precursors).

Clitoroplasty, especially in an adult, is a rare procedure. The goals of clitoroplasty are to achieve a normal genital appearance and to preserve sensation with a satisfactory sexual response [6]. Surgical interventions for this condition present a series of reservations, from patients to practitioners, based on the fears of nerve destruction and loss of sensibility affecting future sexual response and orgasm achievement. As described by Hendren and Crawford [7], reduction clitoroplasty is used to be the most widely accepted and practiced surgical management for the treatment of clitoromegaly since it would maximize clitoral esthetic, while preserving potential sexual function through neurovascular conservation [8]. Surgery for clitoral reduction has been practiced for over half a century to allow female sex assignment and rearing in selected patients [9], mostly infants presenting with genitalia ambigua. A surgical method for the correction of clitoromegaly was first described in 1937 by Young [10], who performed a clitorectomy on a child with congenital adrenal hyperplasia [6]. Until the 1960s, clitorectomy or clitoral amputation was widely accepted as standard treatment [11]. Techniques of reduction and relocation of the clitoris (and recession) were introduced in 1961 by Lattimer [12] and in 1970 by Randolph and Hung [13]. Patients who were submitted to these procedures as infants further reported painful erection when fully grown [9].

The dorsal nerves of the clitoris (DNC) are the primary somatosensory nerves mediating sensation from the clitoris, and its function and integrity are critical for sexual function. According to Poppas, the average size of the dorsal nerves found on their study was 735 μm [8], while O'Connel and Ginger reported 2 mm [14–16]. More recently, Kelling found that DNC were larger than expected (2.0–3.2 mm) when they dissected the clitorises from 10 fresh cadaver specimens [17]. Understanding the anatomical course of the dorsal nerves of the clitoris is therefore important for any female genital cosmetic surgery (FCGS), mainly those which include clitoral hood reduction or plastic, but *mostly* for clitoroplasty. The anatomical location of these nerves has been described in fetal [18] and adult specimen [16, 17, 19]. Dorsal nerve neuroanatomy is comparable in adult and fetal patients, so that surgical technique remains identical at all ages [8]. According to literature, the nerves originate from beneath the pubic bone, inferior to the inferior pubic ramus, and travel along the superior/posterior edge of the clitoral crus. At the angle of the clitoral body, inferior to the pubic symphysis, the DNC enter the deep component of the suspensory ligament, which attaches the clitoral body to the pubic symphysis, forming two large bundles that fanned out laterally on the corporal bodies where the two crural bodies joined to form the single

Fig. 16.1 Findings after careful dissection of the clitoral hood separating the external leaflet from the internal one: white arrow showing the suspensory ligament, black arrows showing the left and right dorsal nerves of the clitoris

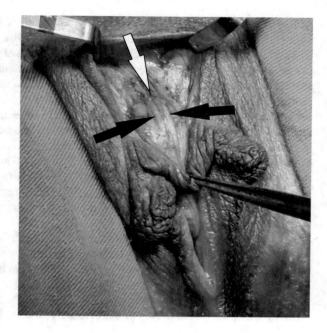

clitoral body with its midline septum. Innervation of the glans clitoris is due to extensive branching as the nerves diverge at the distal end of the corporal bodies (Fig. 16.1).

The nerves course dorsally along the shaft of the clitoris, lying between the clitoral fascia and the tunica albuginea, and happened to be found on varying positions along the clitoral circumference, ranging from 10 to 2 o'clock positions, with a consensus that the 12 o'clock position and the area between the 5 and 7 o'clock positions are free of any nerves [16–19]. It is also expected that in hypertrophied clitoris the dorsal nerves might be found in a more lateral position [8], allowing a safe dorsal midline suture at 12 o'clock position when performing a clitoropexy.

Surgical Technique

This clitoroplasty technique is my personal choice when first treating patients presenting with clitoral hypertrophy, excessive exposure of the glans, or clitoral ptosis with long/hypertrophic/exuberant/redundant hood. Other procedures can be performed along with the clitoropexy, such as labia minora reduction labiaplasty, labia majora reduction labiaplasty, labia majora augmentation by autologous fat transplantation, other plastic surgeries, etc.

The surgical technique consists of a single-stage procedure based on a modification of the technique described by Fuertes Lanzuela [20], preserving the dorsal neurovascular bundle. My equipment of choice for incisions and dissections in labiaplasty, clitoral hood reduction, and clitoroplasty or clitoropexy is a 4 MHz High Frequency Scalpel WAVETRONIC™ (Loktal Medical Electronics Ind. & Com. Ltd., São Paulo—SP, Brazil) due to the hair-thin electrode tip with which I can perfectly visualize and control the exact position and depth of incision and dissection while operating. The procedure is performed in the high dorsal lithotomy position under spinal anesthesia and sedation in order to offer the patients the best experience in terms of comfort and higher grade of refinement in their surgical results. In this technique, the clitoral hood is marked and incised on a line that starts at the transition of the mucosa to the skin and extends about 3 cm down either side of the hood (Fig. 16.2), creating two leaflets, one external and one internal, exposing the suspensory ligament and clitoral body. The mucosa of the prepuce is kept attached to the clitoris, allowing a more physiologic contact with the glans and leaving a free clitoral hood skin flap to be trimmed according to the needs for covering the glans.

Careful dissection proceeds toward the pubic bone through the superficial component of the suspensory ligament (Fig. 16.3), preserving its attachment to the tunica albuginea of the clitoral body in order to maintain the integrity of the neural branches that run through it.

Clitoropexy is achieved by three stitches sutured at the 12, 4, and 8 o'clock positions, avoiding the dorsal nerves of the clitoris, which are located at the 10(11) and

Fig. 16.2 The incision line is done on the transition between the skin of the clitoral hood and the mucosa of the prepuce

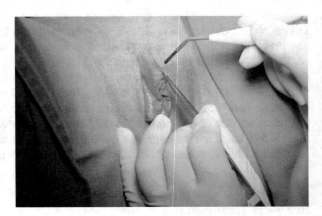

Fig. 16.3 Careful dissection though the superficial component of the suspensory ligament preserving the neural branches underneath

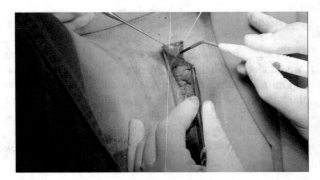

1(2) o'clock positions. The first suture is positioned in the midline (Fig. 16.4), immediately posterior to the prepuce, connecting the clitoral body to the periosteum of the pubis with a 2-0 Prolene™ suture (Ethicon, Somerville, NJ, USA)—bringing the glans to a more inner-upward location—clitoropexy (Fig. 16.5).

The second and third stitches are sutured on either lateral-inferior side of the clitoral body, in order to rotate down the glans, balancing its exposition angle to mimic a more natural appearance. The suspensory ligament is reconnected using 4-0 Vicryl™ sutures (Ethicon, Somerville, NJ, USA), the excess skin from the clitoral hood is trimmed (Fig. 16.6), and its end is sutured to the end of the prepuce with 5-0 Vicryl™ suture (Ethicon, Somerville, NJ, USA) (Fig. 16.7).

Fig. 16.4 The first suture of the clitoropexy is positioned in the midline, immediately posterior to the prepuce, connecting the clitoral body to the periosteum of the pubis

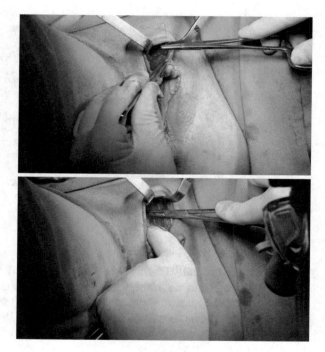

Fig. 16.5 The midline suture allows the glans to be pulled up to a more inner-upward location

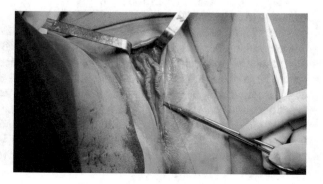

Fig. 16.6 The excess skin from the clitoral hood is trimmed and its end is sutured to the end of the prepuce

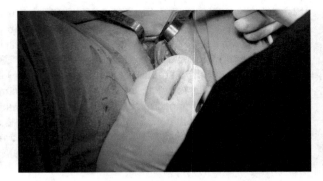

Fig. 16.7 Final refinement: suturing the skin from the clitoral hood to the mucosa of the prepuce

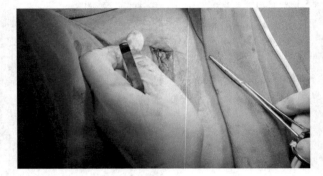

Postoperative Care

The patients are generally discharged on the same day after recovering full control and sensibility of the lower limbs, mainly when operated on the early morning. Pain is one of the most concerning symptoms for patients after surgery; nevertheless, it is well tolerated and/or conducted after this procedure. We usually prescribe keto-profen 200 mg orally once a day for the first 5 days and other analgesics as needed, depending on the discomfort. If the patient still presents with mild pain, we start with dipyrone/acetaminophen 500 mg orally 4–6 h. For moderate pain, we prescribe ketorolac trometamol 10 mg orally 6–8 h. For severe pain (I would say: "very rare, be aware!"), we prescribe codeine 30 mg + acetaminophen 500 mg orally 4–6 h. In this particular case, look for any other possible cause of severe pain rather than only trust it as a personal characteristic for that specific patient: you may find it. Icing should be done when first available for about 30 min, 4–6 times/day, for the first 3 or 4 days after surgery. Hygiene is advised with one or two times rinse, with only water and mild soap, during shower. Excessive cleaning is more harmful than help-ful. Clothing should be loose (dresses and skirts), and underwear should not be too tight or too loose. Avoid jeans, pants, tights, etc. After 3–5 days from surgery, all patients may return to their daily activities and are able to resume sexual relations and physical exercises after 45 days. We schedule a first revision consultation on the 7th to 15th day after surgery, and the follow-up routine comprehends a 12-month period, with scheduled revisions on months 1, 3, 6, and 12 postop to keep a close eye on the patient.

Results

In this chapter, we present the cases of four patients with different clinical presentations from different etiologies to illustrate the wide range of indications for our technique.

In order to satisfactorily compare the postoperative result with the preoperative case, all patients had their photographic documentation according to my own personal standards, which include several caption angles, here simplified by only two of them: one frontal (captured at 15° from the horizontal axis) and one lateral ("left superior oblique position," captured at 45° from all axes) which I call the *Kruse incidence*, that gives a closer and better idea of the three-dimensional shape for the clitoral hood and clitoris and their protruding hypertrophic state.

Patient A, a 25-year-old patient complaining of clitoromegaly, labia minora hypertrophy, labia majora hypotrophy, and overexposed introitus (mainly due to exogenous testosterone intake) was submitted to clitoropexy, clitoral hoodplasty (clitoral hood reduction), labia minora reduction labiaplasty, and labia majora augmentation by autologous fat transplantation (Figs. 16.8 and 16.9).

Patient B, a 32-year-old patient complaining of clitoromegaly, clitoral hood skin redundance, and labia minora hypertrophy mainly due to exogenous oxandrolone intake, was submitted to clitoropexy, clitoral hoodplasty (clitoral hood reduction), and labia minora reduction labiaplasty (Figs. 16.10 and 16.11).

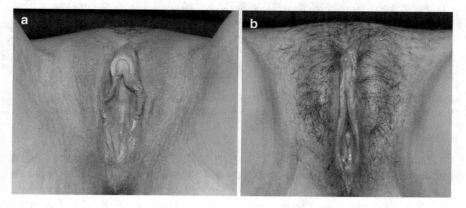

Fig. 16.8 Patient A (25 years old)—clitoropexy, clitoral hood reduction, labia minora reduction labiaplasty, and labia majora augmentation by autologous fat transplantation of 6 mL on each side (12 mL total). (**a**) Preoperative frontal view. (**b**) One-month postoperative frontal view

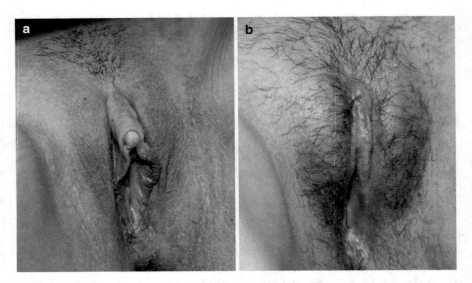

Fig. 16.9 Patient A (25 years old)—clitoropexy, clitoral hood reduction, labia minora reduction labiaplasty, and labia majora augmentation by autologous fat transplantation of 6 mL on each side (12 mL total). (**a**) Preoperative lateral view. (**b**) One-month postoperative lateral view

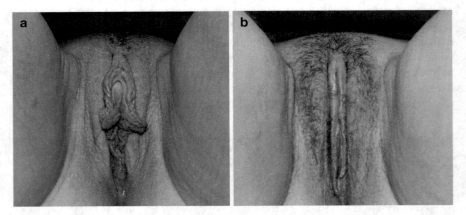

Fig. 16.10 Patient B (32 years old)—clitoropexy, clitoral hood reduction, and labia minora reduction labiaplasty. (**a**) Preoperative frontal view. (**b**) One-month postoperative frontal view

Patient C, a 26-year-old patient who was previously submitted to a botched labia minora and clitoral hood reduction surgery and afterwards decided to underwent an exogenous steroid intake, presented complaining of a detached hypertrophic glans and clitoris overexposure. The patient was submitted to bilateral frenula reconstruction, clitoropexy, clitoral hoodplasty (clitoral hood reconstruction), and labia majora augmentation by autologous fat transplantation (Figs. 16.12 and 16.13).

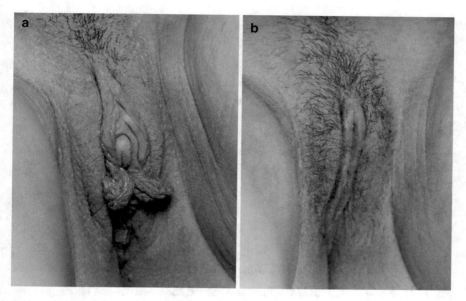

Fig. 16.11 Patient B (32 years old)—clitoropexy, clitoral hood reduction, and labia minora reduction labiaplasty. (**a**) Preoperative lateral view. (**b**) One-month postoperative lateral view

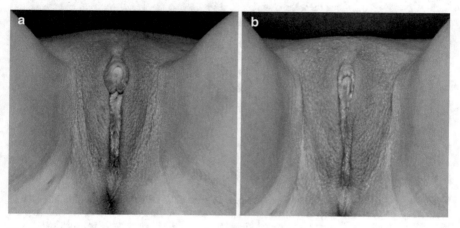

Fig. 16.12 Patient C (26 years old)—clitoropexy, clitoral hood reduction and labia majora augmentation by autologous fat transplantation of 8 mL on each side (16 mL total). (**a**) Preoperative frontal view. (**b**) Three-month postoperative frontal view

Patient D, a 58-year-old patient previously submitted to a labia minora and clitoral hood reduction approximately 25 years before, presented complaining of an exuberant clitoral hood, labia minora asymmetry, and labia majora hypotrophy. The patient was submitted to clitoropexy, clitoral hoodplasty (clitoral hood reduction),

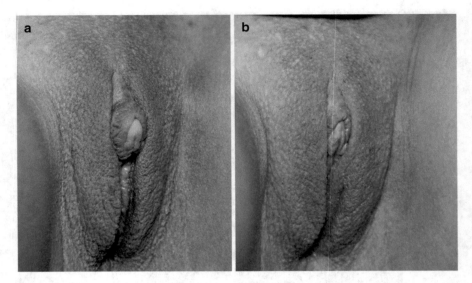

Fig. 16.13 Patient C (26 years old)—clitoropexy, clitoral hood reduction and labia majora augmentation by autologous fat transplantation of 8 mL on each side (16 mL total). (**a**) Preoperative lateral view. (**b**) Three-month postoperative lateral view

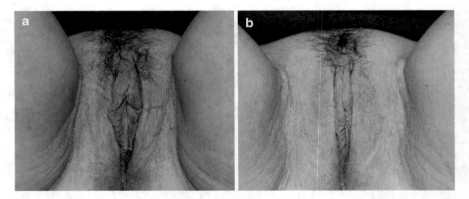

Fig. 16.14 Patient D (58 years old)—clitoropexy, clitoral hood reduction, labia minora reduction labiaplasty, and labia majora augmentation by autologous fat transplantation of 8.5 mL on each side (17 mL total). (**a**) Preoperative frontal view. (**b**) Six-month postoperative frontal view

and labia majora augmentation by autologous fat transplantation (Figs. 16.14 and 16.15).

Clitoral orgasm has been achieved in all patients without pain. Hypersensitivity of the glans prior to surgery remitted after clitoropexy in all patients who had it. None of the patients reported any loss of sensitivity in the clitoris. All patients were satisfied with the aesthetical and functional results of their procedures.

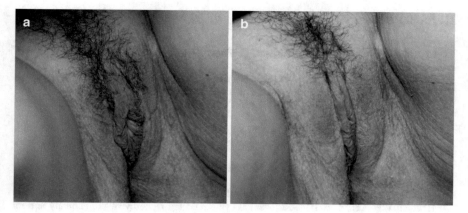

Fig. 16.15 Patient D (58 years old)—clitoropexy, clitoral hood reduction, labia minora reduction labiaplasty, and labia majora augmentation by autologous fat transplantation of 8.5 mL on each side (17 mL total). (**a**) Preoperative lateral view. (**b**) Six-month postoperative lateral view

Complications

The most common complication with this procedure is bleeding and/or hematoma, mainly on the early postoperative period (one particular case presented with arterial bleeding surprisingly on the 18th postoperative day). Other possible complications are wound dehiscence and rupture of the internal points of suture that sustain the clitoropexy, mostly when the patients return to their full activities earlier than recommended (very frequent among these patients, unfortunately). The most feared complication in plastics—and every surgical specialty—is necrosis. Two main causes are ischemia, due to devascularization or arterial strangulation during dissection or repositioning the clitoris, and burns due to excessive energy applied when incising, dissecting, or coagulating vessels, causing tissue burning (arterial, venous, soft tissue, or skin).

Summary

With this technique we believe to succeed on achieving a normal genital appearance while preserving sensation with a satisfactory sexual and orgasmic response. The intercurrences that may happen are inherent to any surgical procedure and are possibly treated without any compromise to the final aesthetic results after all. With all that being said, we conclude that this is a safe and easily reproducible technique, allowing a satisfactory option for treating adult patients with clitoral hypertrophy without compromising the clitoral function.

References

1. Horejsi J. Acquired clitoral enlargement: diagnosis and treatment. Ann N Y Acad Sci. 1997;816:369–72.
2. Oyama IA, Steinberg AC, Holzberg AS, Maccarone JL. Reduction clitoroplasty: a technique for debulking the enlarged clitoris. J Pediatr Adolesc Gynecol. 2004;17:393–5.
3. Tagatz GE, Kopher RA, Nagel TC, Okagaki T. The clitoral index: a bioassay of androgenic stimulation. Obstet Gynecol. 1979;54(5):562–4.
4. Puppo V. Anatomy and physiology of the clitoris, vestibular bulbs, and labia minora with a review of the female orgasm and the prevention of female sexual dysfunction. Clin Anat. 2013;26:134–52.
5. Copcu E, Aktas A, Sivrioglu N, Copcu O, Oztan Y. Idiopathic isolated clitoromegaly: a report of two cases. Reprod Health. 2004;1:4.
6. Sayer RA, Deutsch A, Hoffman MS. Clitoroplasty. Obstet Gynecol. 2007;110(2 II):523–5.
7. Hendren WH, Crawford JD. Androgenital syndrome: the anatomy of the anomaly and its repair – some new concepts. J Pediatr Surg. 1969;4:49.
8. Poppas DP, Hochsztein AA, Baergen RN, Lloyd E, Chen J, Felsen D. Nerve sparing ventral clitoroplasty preserves dorsal nerves in congenital adrenal hyperplasia. J Urol. 2007;178:1802–6. discussion 1806
9. Lean WL, Hutson JM, Deshpande AV, Grover S. Clitoroplasty: past, present and future. Pediatr Surg Int. 2007;23:289–93.
10. Young HH. Genital abnormalities, hermaphroditism and related adrenal disease. Baltimore, MD: Williams and Wilkins; 1937. p. 103–5.
11. Allen LE, Hardy BE, Churchill BM. The surgical management of the enlarged clitoris. J Urol. 1982;128:351–4.
12. Lattimer JK. Relocation and recession of the enlarged clitoris with preservation of the glans: an alternative to amputation. J Urol. 1961;86:113–6.
13. Randolph JG, Hung W. Reduction clitoroplasty in females with hypertrophied clitoris. J Pediatr Surg. 1970;5:224–31.
14. O'Connel HE, Hutson JM, Anderson CR, Plenter RP. Anatomical relationship between urethra and clitoris. J Urol. 1998;159:1892.
15. O'Connel HE, Sanjeevan, Hutson JM. Anatomy of the clitoris. J Urol. 2005;174:1189.
16. Ginger VAT, Cold CJ, Yang CC. Surgical anatomy of the dorsal nerve of the clitoris. Neurol Urodyn. 2011;30:412–6.
17. Kelling JA, Erickson CR, Pin J, Pin PG. Anatomical dissection of the dorsal nerve of the clitoris. Aesthet Surg J. 2020;40(5):541–7.
18. Baskin LS, Erol A, Li YW, Liu WH, Kurzrock E, Cunha GR. Anatomical studies of the human clitoris. J Urol. 1999;162:1015.
19. Marino VD, Lepidi H. Anatomic study of the clitoris and the bulbo-clitoral organ, vol. 9. Switzerland: Springer International Publishing; 2014.
20. Fuertes Lanzuela S, Cartagena Sanchez P. Hiperplasia suprarrenal congénita virilizante. Retroposición del clítoris (versus amputación). Cir Plas Iberolatinoam. 1985;11(1):65–70.

Chapter 17
Quality Training in Gyn-Aesthetics

Rafael Sánchez-Borrego ⓘ, Manuel Sánchez-Prieto ⓘ,
and Pablo Gonzalez-Isaza

Introduction

Regenerative and functional gynecology (gyn-aesthetics), a relatively new, dynamic, and expanding field, holds the promise of enhancing sexual performance and functional and aesthetic enhancement of the genitourinary area of women. The lack of regulation and consensus has not prevented it from acquiring a major role in recent years.

There has been an avalanche of publicity about labiaplasty and other cosmetic vulvovaginal surgical procedures. Some call it "designer laser vaginoplasty," "vaginal rejuvenation," "revirgination," or "G-shot." These procedures and their credibility have sensitized the medical community and the general population. The medicalization (and, by extension, surgery) of sexual behavior, where pharmacological and surgical interventions are promoted to improve sexual pleasure, has even been denounced. It has even been evaluated whether female genital cosmetic surgery (FGCS), referring to procedures that change the structure and appearance of

R. Sánchez-Borrego (✉)
Gynecology and Obstetrics Department, DIATROS Woman's Clinic, Barcelona, Spain

Functional and Cosmetic Gynecology and Cosmetic Genital Surgery, Degree University, Barcelona, Spain
e-mail: rschez.borrego@diatros.com

M. Sánchez-Prieto
Gynecology and Obstetrics Department, Dexeus University Institute, Barcelona, Spain
e-mail: mansan@dexeus.com

P. Gonzalez-Isaza
Obstetrics and Gynecology Urogynecology Minimally Invasive Surgery Functional Cosmetic and Regenerative Gynecology, Hospital Universitario San Jorge/Liga contra el Cancer, Pereira, Madrid, Spain

© The Author(s), under exclusive license to Springer Nature Switzerland AG 2023
P. Gonzalez-Isaza, R. Sánchez-Borrego (eds.), *Topographic Labiaplasty*, https://doi.org/10.1007/978-3-031-15048-7_17

healthy female genitalia for nonmedical reasons, violates the Female Genital Mutilation Act of 2003, in light of CPS guidance issued in 2019 and literature regarding the motivations of women seeking FGCS and its effectiveness [1]. In fact, the ethics and propriety of the procedures themselves and, above all, the training of many of the physicians who perform these procedures have been questioned.

Gyn-aesthetic training should strive for the comprehensive teaching of all medically indicated procedures. However, above all, and for the benefit of women's health, practices and education must be standardized.

Functional Area

Gyn-aesthetics needs to be seen as an independent functional area in the medical community. This functional area includes teams of professionals who have similar skills and experience and who, together, respond to and satisfy the needs of the area in question.

It has been suggested that gynecologists should be the only professionals who perform any technique on the genital area [2]; however, when viewed from a functional area approach, it is feasible for any physician who knows genitourinary pathophysiology and is adequately trained in vulvar and vaginal anatomy to perform the planned surgical procedures. On the other hand, patients should be aware of the training and professional experience of the doctors who treat them.

Ideally, as in most functional areas, training should be provided by a *multidisciplinary team* of healthcare professionals, including physicians, surgeons, sexologists, psychologists, psychotherapists, and physical therapists. Many medical specialties can actively contribute to this functional area. These specialties include cosmetic medicine, general surgery, plastic surgery, gynecology, urology, and dermatology. These specialists already perform cosmetic procedures and reconstructive work and can actively contribute to advancing training in this field.

Training Guidelines

Since the list of surgical and nonsurgical options is extensive and is flourishing with new innovations, having representative professionals with different backgrounds allows for broader options for women and improved physician ability to select the best treatment for patients. In addition, the multidisciplinary team will also be able to continually evaluate and review the educational content and results.

The current terminology used to describe cosmetic gynecologic procedures includes many nondescriptive, proprietary, or informal names, contributing to substantial ambiguity about their specific goals and techniques. Members of the International Urogynecological Association (IUGA) and the American Urogynecologic Society (AUGS) have developed a terminology report for elective cosmetic gynecology procedures, anatomic classification, outcome metrics, and reporting of complications [3].

Understanding Genitourinary Pathophysiology

Menopause and aging are associated with reduced levels of sex steroid hormones, resulting in physiological, biological, and clinical changes in vulvovaginal tissues that contribute to urogenital atrophy, a chronic and progressive condition. There is a potential negative impact on all urogenital tissue quality including the vulva, vagina, bladder, and urethra [4].

Vulvovaginal health care has always been closely linked to understanding and correcting hormonal disorders that cause vulvovaginal atrophy (VVA)/dryness and more problematic situations such as sexual dysfunction, postcoital bleeding, and recurrent urinary tract infections [5]. The predominant connection among the vaginal microbiome, mucosal immunity, and urogenital atrophy occurs through the influential actions of hormones [6]. Vaginal innervation is also strongly influenced by the hormonal milieu, with altered estrogen levels impacting sympathetic, parasympathetic, and sensory nerves [7]. Therefore, it is plausible that symptoms such as hyperalgesia, dyspareunia, and vaginal dryness are due, at least in part, to a higher density of sensory and sympathetic afferents caused by decreased estrogen levels [8]. In addition to estrogens, androgens also contribute to the genitourinary health of women, given the necessary precursors for estrogen biosynthesis and the deficiency in hormones both with aging and after menopause [9, 10]. This is a compelling justification for expanding knowledge about the role of hormones in female genital cosmetic specialists.

Understanding the Mechanisms of Action of Therapies Used

It is essential to know how a drug, other substances, or nonpharmacological intervention produces an effect in the body. For example, the mechanism of action of a drug could be the way it modifies a specific target in the cell, that is, an enzyme or a function such as cell multiplication. Knowing the mechanism of action provides information on the safety of the drug and its effects on the body. In addition, it may help identify the appropriate dose of the drug and the patients who are most likely to respond to treatment.

Estrogens are the gold standard of urogenital atrophy therapy. Estrogen reduces vaginal pH, increases subepithelial capillary growth, thickens the epithelium, increases the level of vaginal secretions, and increases the transvaginal potential difference, reflecting a restoration of normal active transport mechanisms in the vaginal epithelium [8]. The effects of estrogen on the female lower urological tract may be mediated by stimulating the growth of the urethral epithelium or by improving the function of the urethral sphincter or pelvic floor, but the observed effects have been variable [11].

Early treatment of VVA symptoms, when they are moderate rather than severe, may be associated with greater benefits from treatment [12]. However, it is possible that the effects of topical estrogens are limited to the vaginal epithelium, causing a maturation of basal cells and a thickening of the epithelial layer without an impact on the vaginal stroma or vascularization [13]. In addition, and since the therapeutic effect of local vaginal estrogen supplementation disappears once treatment is discontinued, therapies are being developed that provide more sustainable relief of urogenital atrophy symptoms.

Energy-based devices include fractionated lasers (carbon dioxide, erbium:YAG, and hybrid technologies) and monopolar radiofrequency devices. These devices work through heat on the vulva or vaginal mucosa, with the intention of promoting re-epithelialization and neovascularization [14]. The mechanism of action is to cause microtrauma to induce collagen formation, angiogenesis, and epithelial thickening, with the objective of remodeling the vaginal tissue from an atrophied to a thickened, glycogen-rich, and well-vascularized state [15]. Heat shock proteins (HSPs) 43, 47, and 70 have been proposed to activate the production of new collagen and other components of the extracellular matrix [16, 17]. Histological findings revealed epithelial atrophy reversal and collagen remodeling of the vaginal wall. Immunohistochemical analysis showed an increase in collagen type III fibers [18]. Debate continues over its efficacy and safety [19, 20].

Biostimulation with autologous growth factors, mainly of platelet origin, represents the possibility of inducing biological activation of the anabolic functions of the fibroblast through signaling agents, in this case from the group of cytokines [21]. This activation entails notable increases in fibroblast populations in the treated areas and the activation of their anabolism, with an overproduction of hyaluronic acid, reticular collagen, and elastin. It also involves the interesting transformation of some fibroblasts into myofibroblasts and neoangiogenesis and neovascularization, with great therapeutic potential [22].

Currently, there is a new modality in town: stem cell therapy and regenerative medicine. Regenerative medicine and regenerative therapies are new terms and indeed new specialties that have exploded in terms of laboratory research and funding. The route to the market has been swift, with therapies on sale for several clinical applications [23]. Adipose-derived stem cells (ADSCs) are a source of adult stem cells within adipose tissue. ADSCs are of great research interest for the regenerative medicine field due to their ease of harvest, proliferation, and differentiation (to adipose tissue) potential, and very favorable immunological properties [24].

Surgical Training

Formal instruction in surgical skills significantly improves the objective competence and perceived confidence of the student [25]. Regular and ongoing exposure to basic education in surgical skills should be emphasized to foster greater interest in surgery and improve proficiency.

It has been widely claimed that reductions in allocated teaching time and the widespread implementation of short-cut teaching methodologies have led to a short-fall in anatomy knowledge among graduating doctors [26]. This decline in knowledge is evident in the failure of anatomy content to prepare graduates for contemporary clinical practice. The implications for postgraduate surgical training are addressed in the numerous extracurricular anatomy courses available to surgical candidates. As the gender revolution and the female genital cosmetic surgery industry flourish, no contemporary anatomy textbook addresses issues of diversification of female genitalia nor gives medical graduates a realistic view of what is normal regarding female genital appearance.

Genital anatomy is more diverse than we previously thought, and there is evidence to suggest that the labia minora with their rich innervation play an important role in sexual arousal and pleasure. Education regarding the wide range of normal genital appearance suffices in most cases to dissolve concerns regarding body self-image [27].

Female cosmetic surgery (genital plastic surgery or vulvovaginal cosmetic surgery) is a rapidly growing field, and with the complexities and nuances of new technologies and procedures, it is undeniable that additional training is needed. It is accepted that, as in other surgical disciplines, various techniques and instrumentation are used in performing these procedures [28]. Surgeons, the marketplace, and ideally evidence-based outcome data will determine the superiority of one method or technique over another [28]. At this time, due to the lack of rigorous clinical or scientific evidence of short-term and long-term efficacy and safety, such procedures cannot yet be supported in the absence of a functional and medical indication [29]. In addition, the demand for surgical correction after "botched labiaplasty" is on the rise. Women whose expectations have not been met by primary surgery are targeted for repeat surgery through online advertising capitalizing on their potentially unchanged motivations [30].

An important consideration in simulations for surgical training is the fidelity or "realism" of the teaching model [25]. Simulation is an effective method to improve results, but it has limitations related to cost and time [31]. It is plausible that more realistic training models offer an improved experience and will enhance practical competence. At selected institutions, access to ultrahigh fidelity tissue (fresh cadaver) is often made available to trainees for simulation and training purposes. The question remains whether high-fidelity models, such as cadaveric tissue, offer an advantage in surgical education and whether attempts should be made to use these materials when they become available for training.

Training in the Use of New Techniques and New Technologies

In teacher training, the incorporation of new regenerative techniques and new technologies that are unknown to most professionals is imperative. Training must not only instruct teachers to understand and use technological equipment; above all, it must also encourage a reflection about the impact on learning and proper use, potential, and limitations of the technique.

Platelet-rich plasma (PRP), or better said platelet-enriched plasma, is obtained from a sample of blood from a patient taken at the time of treatment and prepared by a process known as differential centrifugation, in which the acceleration force is adjusted to sediment certain cellular components based on different specific weights [22]. In a pilot study, 47 postmenopausal women with VVA were included, with a treatment protocol of 2 A-PRP injection sessions with an interval of 1 month [32]. Response was assessed using the Vaginal Health Index (VHI) and the Vulvovaginal Symptom Questionnaire (VSQ) at baseline and 1 month after the last session. Side effects were also evaluated. Autologous platelet-rich plasma injection was found to be safe and effective as a minimally invasive monotherapy for postmenopausal VVA without a history of breast cancer and thus for vulvovaginal rejuvenation [32]. Since there are many ways to prepare PRP, it is necessary to know the different techniques for its implementation.

Enthusiasm for the potential of cell-based therapies is often directed at clinical needs where currently available medical and pharmacological solutions are unsatisfactory or imperfect. This is a new regenerative approach based on adipose-derived stem cell grafting. However, the need for all patients to undergo liposuction to isolate adipose-derived stem cells means that the process still requires surgery, which has a significant impact on the health system and the lifestyle of patients.

Photobiomodulation therapy has been proposed as an alternative for use in managing urogenital atrophy and stress urinary incontinence (SUI) [33]. The introduction of energy-based devices in this functional area also adds to the debate on the appropriate integration of gyn-aesthetic procedures, as well as adequate training in the use of these devices. Clinicians should be aware of the differences among types of lasers, as well as the research and evidence for the safety and efficacy of individual lasers, including the specific clinical indication, target tissue (e.g., skin, animal model, epithelium), and energy levels used for treatment parameters. Most of the research has been published using microablative fractional CO_2 lasers (wavelength 10,600 nm) and nonablative photothermal erbium:YAG lasers (wavelength of 2940 nm) [34]. However, there are more than 15 LASER companies in the market, encouraged in part by less stringent health agencies' criteria for new medical devices compared with drug approval.

The US Food and Drug Administration (FDA) issued a warning in July 2018 about performing unapproved vaginal cosmetic procedures related to menopause, urinary incontinence, or sexual function [35]. This is especially true since one of the proposed ways of operating this device is by stimulating fibrosis [36]. In any other body system, the stimulation of fibrosis can cause scarring. We do not know if this is the case with these devices. If it is, its application could lead to a worsening of bodily function, especially regarding dyspareunia. We clearly need more information.

Where Are We Going? Should We Go?

Unlike other scientific events, gyn-aesthetics did not start in academic centers with organized programs. It began with largely self-study training, sometimes following the path of trial and error and conducting training on patients whom we put at risk while we learned. We have even introduced an energy-based apparatus as a surgical tool to perform these types of procedures [37].

Specialized and dedicated training is required in the area of female genital cosmetics. However, there is still debate about the suitability required to consider a doctor "competent" in the different medical or surgical techniques in that area. Options include self-guided learning with continuing medical education, a short mentoring period, or a structured postgraduate training program (expert, specialist, or master's degree). We believe that the latter is the best option.

Learn to Be "Critical" of Information

Most of the wealth of information in the medical literature about gyn-aesthetics reflects clinical and scientific advances, but most of it is expert opinion. We must be "critical" and not interpret that the information dictates an exclusive course of treatment or procedure to be followed. It would be worrisome if we ignored the peer-reviewed clinical trial data and simply believed research articles that appear in basic science journals or nonindexed journals. This would incline us to immediately apply these findings in the clinical setting.

It is undeniable that, in today's cosmetic environment, many treatment modalities are carried out despite the absence of peer-reviewed evidence or clinical reviews to support their efficacy. Many therapies are widely advertised and promoted on social media, and after a period, the therapy is accepted without any preexisting evidence of direct benefit or any data on complications [24].

Unfortunately, the female genital cosmetic area has a poor track record in introducing therapies with little evidence base. In a functional area of medicine where outcome measures can be very difficult to determine successfully, many treatments have gained a foothold in the arsenal from minimal and superficial research.

Commercial pressures often take precedence over normal processes that should await the conclusions of peer-reviewed outcome studies. In many situations, these studies are not available at all. Many therapeutic nonsurgical gestures and modalities are introduced directly to the market, bypassing any form of regulation or evidence, and can be offered free to patients [24]. A lack of research and a lack of uniformity, even in terms of the mode of administration, often make it difficult to discover the causality of complications [24].

Controversies in Training

The principles of medical ethics dictate the consideration of autonomy, nonmalefi-cence, beneficence, and justice in the treatment of patients [38]. Any procedure that is more likely to cause harm than good (*primum non nocere*) is unethical.

Although there are discrepancies as to whether gyn-aesthetics is appropriate, there is consensus that certain procedures have not been tested or have such poten-tial risk without proven benefit that they should not be performed at all [28]. "No-go" procedure lists include clitoral unhooding, G-spot amplification, "revirginification" in any form, vulvar recontouring with autologous fat, and so-called "O-shot" injections of PRP that are touted as augmenting the sexual experi-ence. However, the debate has not been resolved, since some believe that it is better to introduce them into the body of doctrine so that if they are indicated, they are carried out with the best possible technique and training.

Certification Program

Classically, training was naturally an exclusive right of official academic institu-tions. Unexpectedly, the emergence of gyn-aesthetic techniques has largely occurred, even for research and innovation, in the private sector rather than the academic sector. As unexpected as it may be, this trend has clear implications for the training of future experts or specialists in this functional area. This new turn in the development of genital aesthetics requires innovative options to optimally meet training obligations.

The objective of a good postgraduate course is to ensure, through a precise selec-tion of theoretical topics and practices ("hands-on," hospital, and patients), that the student is able to adequately diagnose the most prevalent pathology of the female genital area while identifying the level of clinical difficulty in handling cases that arise in daily practice, trying to train him for the management of those that are not complex or advanced cases, and providing him with the knowledge to defer to other experts or specialists. In an academic environment, the collaboration of specialists from different fields around the aesthetics and functional pathology of the female genitalia would provide these postgraduates with a greater wealth in continued medical training.

Summary

The modalities of training in gyn-aesthetic—length of training, theoretical curricu-lum, methods of ensuring competence, and certification processes—differ greatly from country to country. The composition of these courses, the number of hours required, and the course content are not something that we as a profession can nec-essarily legislate, but our purpose is to stimulate a peer group to agree on acceptable standards of care and training requirements. We anticipate that such requirements will specifically include training in sexual medicine sufficient to enable the cosmetic genital surgical physician to assess the sexual health of his or her patient and be able to discover sexual dysfunction that can be disguised with a surgical solution.

The collaboration, in an academic environment, of specialists from different fields around the aesthetics and functional pathology of the female genitalia, would provide these postgraduate courses with a greater richness in continuing medical education.

The objective of a good postgraduate course is to seek, through a precise selection of theoretical issues and practices ("hands-on," hospital, and patients), that the student is able to properly diagnose the most prevalent pathology of the female genital sphere, while identifying the level of clinical difficulty in the management of cases that are presented in daily practice, trying to enable it for the management of those who are not included within complex or advanced cases, but providing knowledge that will allow you to guide an appropriate therapeutic approach by other experts or specialists.

To perform any genital cosmetic procedure, surgeons should be adequately trained and experienced and be clinically competent to perform the procedure [39, 40]. Physicians performing these procedures are expected to have a broad familiarity with appearance and function, as well as the ability to manage complications.

Considerable efforts must be made to standardize this training, even in the difficult times that we are living with this pandemic [41]. This harmonization effort should be based on the development of a detailed program that describes the scope of training in this functional area [41]. This is embodied in our specialization course/postgraduate course in aesthetic and functional gynecology and cosmetic genital surgery of women, which we developed with the University of Barcelona.

References

1. Gaffney-Rhys R. Female genital cosmetic surgery: legitimate refinement or illegal mutilation? Eur J Health Law. 2021;28(3):244–62. https://doi.org/10.1163/15718093-BJA10046.
2. Pauls RN. We are the correct physicians to treat women requesting labiaplasty. Am J Obstet Gynecol. 2014;211(3):218–218.e1. https://doi.org/10.1016/j.ajog.2014.06.019.
3. Developed by the Joint Writing Group of the International Urogynecological Association and the American Urogynecologic Society. Joint report on terminology for cosmetic gynecology. Int Urogynecol J. 2022; https://doi.org/10.1007/s00192-021-05010-7.
4. Tan O, Bradshaw K, Carr BR. Management of vulvovaginal atrophy-related sexual dysfunction in postmenopausal women: an up-to-date review. Menopause. 2012;19(1):109–17. https://doi.org/10.1097/gme.0b013e31821f92df.
5. Iqbal S, Akkour K, Bano B, Hussain G, Elhelow MKKA, Al-Mutairi AM, Aljasim BSK. Awareness about vulvovaginal aesthetics procedures among medical students and health professionals in Saudi Arabia. Rev Bras Ginecol Obstet. 2021;43(3):178–84. https://doi.org/10.1055/s-0041-1725050.
6. Lillemon JN, Karstens L, Nardos R, Garg B, Boniface ER, Gregory WT. The impact of local estrogen on the urogenital microbiome in genitourinary syndrome of menopause: a

randomized-controlled trial. Female Pelvic Med Reconstr Surg. 2022; https://doi.org/10.1097/SPV.0000000000001170.

7. Mónica Brauer M, Smith PG. Estrogen and female reproductive tract innervation: cellular and molecular mechanisms of autonomic neuroplasticity. Auton Neurosci. 2015;187:1–17. https://doi.org/10.1016/j.autneu.2014.11.009.

8. Sánchez-Borrego R, Manubens M, Navarro MC, Cancelo MJ, Beltrán E, Duran M, Orte T, Baquedano L, Palacios S, Mendoza N, Spanish Menopause Society. Position of the Spanish Menopause Society regarding vaginal health care in postmenopausal women. Maturitas. 2014;78(2):146–50. https://doi.org/10.1016/j.maturitas.2014.03.003.

9. Palacios S. Expression of androgen receptors in the structures of vulvovaginal tissue. Menopause. 2020;27(11):1336–42. https://doi.org/10.1097/GME.0000000000001587.

10. Simon JA, Goldstein I, Kim NN, Davis SR, Kellogg-Spadt S, Lowenstein L, Pinkerton JV, Stuenkel CA, Traish AM, Archer DF, Bachmann G, Goldstein AT, Nappi RE, Vignozzi L. The role of androgens in the treatment of genitourinary syndrome of menopause (GSM): International Society for the Study of Women's Sexual Health (ISSWSH) expert consensus panel review. Menopause. 2018;25(7):837–47. https://doi.org/10.1097/GME.0000000000001138.

11. Chen YY, Su TH, Lau HH. Estrogen for the prevention of recurrent urinary tract infections in postmenopausal women: a meta-analysis of randomized controlled trials. Int Urogynecol J. 2021;32(1):17–25. https://doi.org/10.1007/s00192-020-04397-z.

12. Palacios S, Panay N, Sánchez-Borrego R, Particco M, Djumaeva S. Earlier treatment of vulvovaginal atrophy in post-menopausal women may improve treatment outcomes. J Gynecol Womens Health. 2019;16(1):555928. https://doi.org/10.19080/JGWH.2019.16.555928.

13. Gaspar A, Brandi H, Gomez V, Luque D. Efficacy of Erbium:YAG laser treatment compared to topical estriol treatment for symptoms of genitourinary syndrome of menopause. Lasers Surg Med. 2017;49(2):160–8. https://doi.org/10.1002/lsm.22569.

14. Tadir Y, Gaspar A, Lev-Sagie A, Alexiades M, Alinsod R, Bader A, Calligaro A, Elias JA, Gambaciani M, Gaviria JE, Iglesia CB, Selih-Martinec K, Mwesigwa PL, Ogrinc UB, Salvatore S, Scollo P, Zerbinati N, Nelson JS. Light and energy based therapeutics for genitourinary syndrome of menopause: consensus and controversies. Lasers Surg Med. 2017;49(2):137–59. https://doi.org/10.1002/lsm.22637.

15. Salvatore S, Leone Roberti Maggiore U, Athanasiou S, Origoni M, Candiani M, Calligaro A, Zerbinati N. Histological study on the effects of microablative fractional CO_2 laser on atrophic vaginal tissue: an ex vivo study. Menopause. 2015;22(8):845–9. https://doi.org/10.1097/GME.0000000000000401.

16. Lukač M, Lozar A, Perhavec T, Bajd F. Variable heat shock response model for medical laser procedures. Lasers Med Sci. 2019;34(6):1147–58. https://doi.org/10.1007/s10103-018-02704-1.

17. Phillips C, Hillard T, Salvatore S, Toozs-Hobson P, Cardozo L. Lasers in gynaecology. Eur J Obstet Gynecol Reprod Biol. 2020;251:146–55. https://doi.org/10.1016/j.ejogrb.2020.03.034.

18. Bretas TLB, Issa MCA, Fialho SCAV, Villar EAG, Velarde LGC, Pérez-López FR. Vaginal collagen I and III changes after carbon dioxide laser application in postmenopausal women with the genitourinary syndrome: a pilot study. Climacteric. 2022;25(2):186–94. https://doi.org/10.1080/13697137.2021.1941850.

19. Filippini M, Porcari I, Ruffolo AF, Casiraghi A, Farinelli M, Uccella S, Franchi M, Candiani M, Salvatore S. CO_2-laser therapy and genitourinary syndrome of menopause: a systematic review and meta-analysis. J Sex Med. 2022;19(3):452–70. https://doi.org/10.1016/j.jsxm.2021.12.010.

20. Pérez-López FR, Varikasuvu SR. Vulvovaginal atrophy management with a laser: the placebo effect or the conditioning Pavlov reflex. Climacteric. 2022;25:323–6. https://doi.org/10.1080/13697137.2022.2050207.

21. Eppley BL, Pietrzak WS, Blanton M. Platelet-rich plasma: a review of biology and applications in plastic surgery. Plast Reconstr Surg. 2006;118(6):147e–59e. https://doi.org/10.1097/01.prs.0000239606.92676.cf.

22. Abu-Ghname A, Perdanasari AT, Davis MJ, Reece EM. Platelet-rich plasma: principles and applications in plastic surgery. Semin Plast Surg. 2019;33(3):155–61. https://doi.org/10.1055/s-0039-1693400.

23. Lane FL, Jacobs S. Stem cells in gynecology. Am J Obstet Gynecol. 2012;207(3):149–56. https://doi.org/10.1016/j.ajog.2012.01.045.
24. Goddard NV, Waterhouse N. Regenerative medicine, stem cell therapies, and platelet-rich plasma: where is the evidence? Aesthet Surg J. 2020;40(4):460–5. https://doi.org/10.1093/asj/sjz317.
25. Blau JA, Shammas RL, Anolik RA, Avashia YJ, Krucoff KB, Zenn MR. Does realism matter? A randomized controlled trial comparing models for medical student suture education. Plast Reconstr Surg Glob Open. 2020;8(4):e2738. https://doi.org/10.1097/GOX.0000000000002738.
26. Hayes JA, Temple-Smith MJ. New context, new content-rethinking genital anatomy in textbooks. Anat Sci Educ. 2022; https://doi.org/10.1002/ase.2173.
27. Kalampalikis A, Michala L. Cosmetic labiaplasty on minors: a review of current trends and evidence. Int J Impot Res. 2021:1–4. https://doi.org/10.1038/s41443-021-00480-1.
28. Halder GE, Iglesia CB, Rogers RG. Controversies in female genital cosmetic surgeries. Clin Obstet Gynecol. 2020;63(2):277–88. https://doi.org/10.1097/GRF.0000000000000519.
29. Shaw D, Allen L, Chan C, Kives S, Popadiuk C, Robertson D, Shapiro J. Guideline No. 423: Female genital cosmetic surgery and procedures. J Obstet Gynaecol Can. 2022;44(2):204–214. e1. https://doi.org/10.1016/j.jogc.2021.11.001.
30. Learner HI, Rundell C, Liao LM, Creighton SM. 'Botched labiaplasty': a content analysis of online advertising for revision labiaplasty. J Obstet Gynaecol. 2020;40(7):1000–5. https://doi.org/10.1080/01443615.2019.1679732.
31. Gosman A, Mann K, Reid CM, Vedder NB, Janis JE. Implementing assessment methods in plastic surgery. Plast Reconstr Surg. 2016;137(3):617e–23e. https://doi.org/10.1097/01.prs.0000479968.76438.27.
32. Saleh DM, Abdelghani R. Clinical evaluation of autologous platelet rich plasma injection in postmenopausal vulvovaginal atrophy: a pilot study. J Cosmet Dermatol. 2022; https://doi.org/10.1111/jocd.14873.
33. Lanzafame RJ, de la Torre S, Leibaschoff GH. The rationale for photobiomodulation therapy of vaginal tissue for treatment of genitourinary syndrome of menopause: an analysis of its mechanism of action, and current clinical outcomes. Photobiomodul Photomed Laser Surg. 2019;37(7):395–407. https://doi.org/10.1089/photob.2019.4618.
34. Arunkalaivanan A, Kaur H, Onuma O. Laser therapy as a treatment modality for genitourinary syndrome of menopause: a critical appraisal of evidence. Int Urogynecol J. 2017;28(5):681–5. https://doi.org/10.1007/s00192-017-3282-y.
35. FDA warns against use of energy-based devices to perform vaginal "rejuvenation" or vaginal cosmetic procedures: FDA safety communication. Date Issued: July 30, 2018.
36. Escribano JJ, González-Isaza P, Tserotas K, Athanasiou S, Zerbinati N, Leibaschoff G, Salvatore S, Sánchez-Borrego R. In response to the FDA warning about the use of photomedicine in gynecology. Lasers Med Sci. 2019;34(7):1509–11. https://doi.org/10.1007/s10103-019-02744-1.
37. González-Isaza P, Lotti T, França K, Sanchez-Borrego R, Tórtola JE, Lotti J, Wollina U, Tchernev G, Zerbinati N. Carbon dioxide with a new pulse profile and shape: a perfect tool to perform labiaplasty for functional and cosmetic purpose. Open Access Maced J Med Sci. 2018;6(1):25–7. https://doi.org/10.3889/oamjms.2018.043.
38. Barone M, Cogliandro A, Persichetti P. Ethics and plastic surgery/what is plastic surgery? Arch Plast Surg. 2017;44(1):90–2. https://doi.org/10.5999/aps.2017.44.1.90.
39. American College of Obstetricians and Gynecologists. The role of the obstetrician-gynecologist in cosmetic procedures. Statement of Policy. Washington, DC: ACOG; 2018.
40. American College of Obstetricians and Gynecologists. Elective female genital cosmetic surgery. ACOG Committee Opinion No. 795. American College of Obstetricians and Gynecologists. Obstet Gynecol. 2020;135(1):e36–42. https://doi.org/10.1097/AOG.0000000000003616.
41. Sánchez-Borrego R, García-Giménez JV, González-Isaza P, Escribano-Tórtola JJ, Sánchez-Prieto M, Leibaschoff GH, Alijotas-Reig J, on behalf of the board of the Specific Postgraduate Diploma 'Functional and Cosmetic Gynecology and Cosmetic Genital Surgery', University of Barcelona, Spain. Gyn-Aesthetic: the 'new normal' after COVID-19. Clin Obstet Gynecol Reprod Med. 2020;6:1–6. https://doi.org/10.15761/COGRM.1000309.

Chapter 18
Ethical-Legal Aspects

David Vasquez Awad

Introduction

In February 2019 I was invited by my good friend and brilliant disciple Pablo González to give a lecture on "ethics in vaginal cosmetic surgery." The first thing I told Pablo is that I am not a specialist in ethics or bioethics. Perhaps the fact that I have been a teacher for many years, a member of the faculty council of a prestigious university, and a full member of the National Academy of Medicine has allowed me to be in close contact with aspects related to bioethics. But what motivated me the most is that I have not only been skeptical in relation to this medical practice, but I have seen in the years of my private and institutional practice so many good and bad results of this practice, that I decided to accept the challenge and the invitation of the respected colleague and agreed to give the lecture. This text is the result of that conference.

Personally, I am not against vaginal cosmetic surgery. I think it is a valuable tool and, like any approach, its proper use depends on the indications, contraindications, and, most importantly, the stripping of the profit motive to provide women with the best option. I always ask my colleagues: Would you propose the same conduct to the patient if she were not a private patient but an institutional one? Hand on heart, the answer to the question will guide the physician as to what is best for the patient.

This chapter seeks that colleagues who perform genital cosmetic surgery have a practical, quick, and simple orientation to do the right thing. It does not pretend to be a treaty (I repeat I am not a specialist in bioethics) on the subject. When we were medical students, we wanted to train ourselves to do the best for our patients. Putting it into practice now that we are doctors is an ethical obligation.

D. V. Awad (✉)
Obstetrics & Gynecology, Epidemiology, National Academy of Medicine, Bogota DC, Colombia

© The Author(s), under exclusive license to Springer Nature Switzerland AG 2023
P. Gonzalez-Isaza, R. Sánchez-Borrego (eds.), *Topographic Labiaplasty*,
https://doi.org/10.1007/978-3-031-15048-7_18

181

Definition and Historical Notes

Ethics is the *ethos*, the principle, the indisputable, independent of person, country, race, social class, profession, environment, or circumstances. It is a concept different from morality and legality. Morality refers more to the act in relation to the sociocultural environment in which the individual develops. For example, in Western countries, for a woman to go to the beach in a bikini is usually, normal, and does not generate any moral questioning. On the contrary, for a woman to go to the beach in a bikini is considered in orthodox Muslim countries an attack of morality, but not to ethics. Legality, in turn, has to do with legal normativity. An act can be legal but not ethical or moral.

Ethics is that part of philosophy that deals with man's obligations to himself, to the environment around him, to his fellow man, and to the present and future of human well-being.

The word ethics comes from the Greek "ethos" which means way of doing or acquiring things, customs, and habits, plus the suffix "ico" which means relative. The word ethics designates above all a philosophical discipline that studies the foundations of morality in its broadest and most sublime expression.

Contemporary ethics carries out its reflections on three different levels [1]:

- Metaethics, interested in the nature, origin, and meaning of basic ethical concepts, that is, ethics itself.
- Normative ethics, the study of which focuses on the search for and interpretation of normative systems with which to lead human beings towards the best possible life.
- Applied ethics, which consists of the interpretation of specific ethical cases and controversies, generally from real life. This is the one that is applied in a practical and daily way to the medical act, which is what motivates us to write this chapter.

Ethics has been present in the very beginnings of philosophy, especially in classical Greece. Philosophers such as Plato (c. 427–347 BC) and his disciple Aristotle (384–322 BC) studied human conduct and the codes that govern it [1].

His reflections can be found in the Platonic dialogues of Gorgias and Phaedo, as well as in his Republic, or in Aristotle's famous Nicomachean Ethics, the first treatise on ethics in history [1].

In the following centuries, throughout the Middle Ages, Christianity imposed its moral vision on practically all fields and knowledge. It defined faith as the ultimate end of human existence and the precepts of conduct as expressed in the biblical Gospels [1].

The role of ethics then was to interpret in a correct way the sacred scriptures, to compose from its truth the Christian way of being. In this period the works of religious thinkers such as St. Augustine (354–430) and Thomas Aquinas (1224–1274) [1] stand out.

The Modern Age and the humanist vision broke with this tradition, both religious and ancient. The need to construct a new ethical model was imposed, one that responded to reason and to the place that, as the center of creation, the human being now occupied in culture [1].

The great modern philosophers such as René Descartes (1596–1650), Baruch Spinoza (1632–1677), and David Hume (1711–1776) dealt with this complex subject. But it was Immanuel Kant (1724–1804) who made the great modern ethical revolution, with his idea of the categorical imperative [1].

The first time the name "medical ethics" appeared was at the beginning of the nineteenth century by Thomas Percival, who published in 1803 a work with the long title: Medical Ethics or a code of institutions and precepts adapted to the professional conduct of physicians and surgeons: (1) in hospital practice, (2) in private or general practice, (3) in relation to pharmacists, and (4) in cases where a knowledge of the law should be required [2].

Percival's medical model is a vivid reflection of the Hippocratic physician as it has been modulated over time. Emphasis is placed on the figure of the prudent and educated doctor, on the gentle man, and on his being a true gentleman. Medical ethics began to be bureaucratized from this time and became "medical etiquette" [2].

It was from the Nuremberg Code, especially its article 1 ("the voluntary consent of the human subject is absolutely essential"), when the gradual appearance of other types of ethical codes of the health professions began on the one hand and, on the other hand, the publication of important documents of a legal and ethical nature, at national and international level, based preferably on the defense and promotion of the dignity of the human person and respect for their fundamental rights. In recent decades, medical codes of ethics have gone hand to hand with the promotion and defense of human rights and could be listed in chronological order [2]:

1. International codes

> Nuremberg Code 1947
> International Code of Medical Ethics 1949–1983
> Geneva Declaration 1948–1994
> Tokyo Declaration 1975
> Asturias Convention on Bioethics 1997
> Tavistock Principles 1997
> Code of Ethical Principles and Conduct 2001-PAHO/WHO
> International Code of Ethics for Occupational Health Professionals 2002-ICOH/CIST
> Universal Declaration of Ethical Principles for Psychologists 2008

2. Codes at European national level

> Principles of European Medical Ethics 1987
> Code of Medical Ethics/Guide of Medical Ethics 2011—Spain
> Codice Deontologico Medico 2014—Italy

Code de Déontologie Médicale 2012—France
Code of Ethics of the Fédération des Médecins Suisses—2015
Code of Ethics of the Ordem dos Medicos 2015—Portugal
Code Déontologie Médicale 2013—Luxembourg
Code de Déontologie Médicale 2014—Belgium

3. Latin American national codes

Code of Ethics 2010—Colegio Médico de México
Code of Bioethics for Health Personnel 2002—Mexico
Code of Ethics and Medical Deontology 2013—Colegio Médico de El Salvador
Code of Ethics 2005—Colegio Médico de Honduras
Code of Ethics 2009—College of Physicians and Surgeons of Guatemala
Code of Medical Ethics of the Dominican Medical Association 2005—Dominican Republic
Code of Medical Ethics 2009—College of Physicians and Surgeons of the Republic of Costa Rica
Draft Reform of the Medical Code of Ethics 2010—Colombia
Code of Medical Ethics 1992—Ecuadorian Medical Federation
Code of Medical Deontology 2003—Venezuelan Medical Federation
Code of Ethics and Medical Deontology 2010—Bolivian Medical Association
Code of Ethics and Deontology 2007—Peruvian Medical Association
Code of Medical Ethics 2010—Brazilian Federal Council of Medicine
Code of Medical Ethics (Yagecero Doctors)
Code of Ethics 2014—Medical College of Uruguay
Code of Ethics 2013—Colegio Médico de Chile
Code of Ethics—Medical Confederation of Argentina
Code of Ethics for the Health Team (second edition-2011)—Asociación Médica Argentina

4. North American national codes

US Department of Health and Human Services—The Belmont Report—1979
Belmont Report: Spanish version (Observatory on Bioethics and Law—Barcelona)
Principles of Medical Ethics (American Medical Association-AMA)—2001
Code of Ethics of the AMC 2004—Canada

5. Nursing deontological codes

Deontological Code of the Spanish Nursing 1989
ICN Code of Ethics for the Nursing Profession 2012

6. Pharmaceutical codes of ethics

Pharmaceutical Code of Ethics 1999
Code of Pharmaceutical Ethics and Deontology of the Pharmaceutical Profession 2001

Branches of Ethics [3]

Ethics is one of the many branches of philosophy, that studies things by their causes of the universe and these branches can be:

- Ethical goals

    It studies the origin and meaning of ethical concepts, as well as metaphysical questions about morality, in particular whether moral values exist independently of human values and whether they are relative, conventional, or absolute.

    Metaethics does not answer questions such as what is "good," but rather what does a person do when he talks about "good" or what are the characteristics of moral language; some problems of metaethics are the problem of being and ought to be, the problem of moral fate, and the question of the existence or non-existence of free will.

- Normative ethics

    Explores possible moral criteria for determining when an action is right and when it is wrong. It looks for general principles that justify normative systems, arguing why certain norms should be adopted. Within normative ethics, there are three main positions:

    - Consequentialism: Holds that the moral worth of an action should be judged solely on the basis of whether its consequences are favorable or unfavorable. Different versions of consequentialism differ; however, about which consequences should be considered relevant in determining the morality or otherwise of an action.
    - Deontology—Argues that there are duties that must be fulfilled, regardless of the favorable or unfavorable consequences they may bring, and that to fulfill these duties is to act morally. For example, taking care of our children is a duty, and it is morally wrong not to do so, even when this may result in great economic benefits.
    - Virtue ethics focuses on the importance of developing good habits of conduct, or virtues, and avoiding bad habits, or vices.

- Applied ethics

    This is the part of ethics that deals with the study of specific, controversial moral issues. For example, some objects of study in applied ethics are induced abortion, euthanasia, and animal rights. Some of these issues are grouped by similarities and studied by sub-disciplines:

    - Bioethics
    - Professional ethics
    - Environmental ethics
    - Military ethics
    - Economic ethics

Bioethics

Scientists and philosophers were surprised with the new situations raised by the intervention, manipulation, and production created by scientific research. To solve problems that afflict people and societies, it is necessary to turn to theology, ethics, and law, in addition to philosophy, in a search to find solutions to conflicts never before faced by the species [4].

Bioethics is the branch of ethics that provides principles in order to suggest the most appropriate behaviors around making fair and prudent decisions about life, human or nonhuman, even touching on what is related to the environment [4]. Principlism argues that there are some general principles discovered in the field of biomedical ethics that should be respected when ethical conflicts arise in research or clinical practice.

Bioethics has the following principles [5]:

1. The interest of man takes precedence over the mere interests of society and science.
2. Interventions in the field of medicine must be carried out according to the rules and duties of the profession.
3. No intervention may be performed on a person without his or her informed consent.
4. Everyone has the right to be informed about his or her health or to withhold such information.
5. National law should develop special provisions to protect the incapable (minors, incapacitated adults, and the mentally ill).
6. In case of emergency, an intervention can be performed without the corresponding consent.
7. The human body or its parts cannot be a source of profit.
8. Sanctions should be established for cases in which these principles are violated.

Plastic Surgery

Vaginal cosmetic surgery may well be framed within the same plastic surgery and can be:

(a) Reconstructive or restorative
(b) Aesthetics or cosmetics

Either of the two should comply with the basic principles of bioethics (principlism), when making the decision to propose a particular procedure by the physician. These principles, in a simple and practical way, are as follows:

1. Beneficence: favoring those who are affected by the action:
   Does the procedure really benefit the patient or not?

2. Non-malice: *Primun non nocere.*

   Prudence is a quality that avoids accidents and mistakes, thus acquiring the ethical virtue of not being evil: *Am I suitable or not?*

3. Autonomy: The patient must have the ability to decide on his own. *To do so, he/she must receive all the information in an eminently ethical environment.*

4. Justice: It describes preferably the relations between social groups, emphasizing equity in the distribution of resources and goods considered common: *In justice, should these procedures be paid for by society or by the individual?*

In summary:

- Benefit:
  Doing things well in order to do good to others.
- Of the less wrong:
  In case of conflict between two wrong, choose the lesser in impact, duration, and extent.
- Informed consent
  Respecting the person's decision-making capability, dignity, and rights. Agree to interventions on others.
- Justice:
  To provide each patient with an adequate level of care to ensure proper health care.

Bioethics Surrounding a Cosmetic Procedure

An aesthetic act, in the framework of ethics, is a good act if it achieves its intended purpose. To qualify it as good, it is necessary to precisely define the purpose which, ultimately, is not to remove, repair, or replace a diseased organ but to improve the quality of the patient's life [6].

The main mistakes—and very serious from the ethical point of view—that are made in the practice of cosmetic surgery (including genital surgery) are as follows [6]:

1. Lack of professionalism and advertising abuses
   Doctors not certified in the specialty, treatments of "wonderful results," without any scientific evidence, which leads many patients to consult and undergo procedures, with undesired results, or bad results. It is common to hear in the stories of these patients, when they ask to a qualified specialist for their opinion, that there was much lack of communication beforehand and very little responsibility afterwards. This includes the famous "Medical Tourism," so much promoted abroad, especially in Spain, the United States, Central America, and the Caribbean.

2. Lack of scientific evidence
   Practicing procedures without having completed all the steps of the scientific method. It should be noted that many adverse effects are only seen months or years after the procedure.

3. False expectations

It is common to offer treatments that appear to be simple, fast, with excellent results, and without complications, "express surgery," which is promoted, especially in foreign patients, who must necessarily return to their countries a few days later, and whose subsequent evolution, with its complications, and results must be assumed by another doctor. This includes the lack of information about the products or technologies used, doses, precautions, interactions, "good manufacturing practices" certificates, contraindications, possible complications, etc. Most of the time these breaches of ethics are due to the fear that this will scare away the patient or rather "the client."

4. Incitement to cosmetic surgery

Here we include the following:

- Profit through offering or advertising expectations of patients
- Deliver results other than what the procedure entails
- Inappropriately stimulating patient expectations
- Promote an image of "perfect (genital) beauty"
- Promoting a misconception that sexuality is necessarily linked to a specific type of "beauty"

Many of these surgeries are unnecessary. I have seen this in my practice on a daily basis. So, it is worth to clarify a few points of what is "unnecessary" in surgery or inside a procedure [7]:

- Unnecessary does not always mean not 100% beneficial.
- Nor does it always imply 100% maleficence.
- Unnecessary does not always equal 100% unnecessary.
- Does not always imply mercantilist intent.
- Exceptionally, it involves a malicious act.
- Unnecessary for some surgeons but not for others.
- The unnecessary of a type of surgery today could be necessary yesterday and even tomorrow.
- The unnecessariness of one type of surgery may be 100% for one institution but not for another.
- Unnecessary can be 100% for one culture and 0% for another.
- Unnecessary by insufficient action, by not acting and by excess.

Adolescents are a particularly sensitive segment of the population, and, for this reason, the *American College of Obstetricians and Gynecologists (ACOG)* issued recommendations in 2016 [7]. According to the *American Society for Aesthetic Plastic Surgery*, overall labiaplasty increased 16% in the United States in 2015. ACOG's four main recommendations are the following [8]:

1. Physicians should acquire adequate knowledge of the nonsurgical options available and the indications for surgical treatment.
2. Adolescents should be informed about the normal differences in anatomy, growth, and development of the breasts and external genitalia.

3. Prior to surgical evaluation, patients should receive appropriate counseling and assessment of their physical and emotional maturity.
4. Physicians should screen for body dysmorphic disorder, which can lead to repeated cosmetic surgical procedures due to dissatisfaction, and should refer patients to mental health professionals when they suspect it.

Conclusion

Vaginal cosmetic surgery has had a growing boom and popularity in recent years, perhaps because of the overwhelming advance of the cult of physical beauty, because of the self-esteem so stimulated in recent times, because of the role that sexuality has been gaining (fortunately) in the concept of quality of life, because of the advent of new technologies, and, undoubtedly, because of the skill that health professionals have been acquiring.

The most important thing is that the professional is sufficiently trained to perform the procedures he offers and, on the other hand, that his actions are governed by the "principlism" of ethics already explained above. *Pimum non nocere*, the old Latin precept, is still fully in force, and the doctor must get rid of the excessive desire for profit and the aggressiveness of the industry that manufactures equipment and supplies, in order to practice medicine with quality and ethics.

References

1. https://concepto.de/etica/#ixzz6WEur7BAo
2. BIOETHICS from ASTURIAS (Blog). Resources and utilities (Tino Quintana).
3. Gaibor JSQ, Macas JLP. Evolución histórica de la ética hasta nuestros días, Revista Caribeña de Ciencias Sociales; September 2018.
4. Hottois G. What is Bioethics? Libraire Philosophique J. VRIN. 6, Place de la Sorbonne. 2017. U. The Forest.
5. Cf. C. DE SOLA LLERA. Zur Struktur der 'Konvention zum Schutz der Menschenwürde und der Menschenrechte im Hinblick auf die Anwendung von Biologie und Medizin: Bioethik-Konvention' des Europarates. Jahrbuch für Wissenschaft und Ethik. 1996;1:190.
6. Jaime A, Armando OP. Some ethical reflections on plastic surgery. Rev Med Clin Condes. 2010;21(1):135–8.
7. Torres VF. Ethics and surgery. Seminar: The current practice of medicine. Mexico, DF: Division of Postgraduate Studies and Research, Faculty of Medicine UNAM.
8. Committee Opinion No. 662. Obstet Gynecol. 2016;127(5):e138–40. https://doi.org/10.1097/AOG.0000000000001441.

Annexes

Informed Consent

Informed Consent for Medical Procedures

Aesthetic Gynecology

I _____ identified
with ID number _____.

I will be performed by Dr. ------------------------identification------------------------
medical record--------------------------------

_____ Labiaplasty/labia reduction (labia minora and/or labia majora).

_____ Reduction of the clitoral hood/reduction of the size of the clitoral hood.

_____ Addressing anatomical variants (accessory folds in labia clitoral hood) and
perineal region.

_____ Injection of filler materials in labia majora or vagina (hyaluronic acid cross-
linked/non-cross-linked platelet-rich plasma and/or growth factors) with aesthetic
and/or functional purposes.

Please read the following information in detail.
I understand:

1. The risks of surgeries can be the following: prolonged or incomplete healing,
   surgical wound opening, irregularities, abnormal scarring, or asymmetries in
   the size of the labia after surgery, infection, painful sexual intercourse, prolonged bleeding among other rare events.
2. The surgical area will be swollen, asymmetric, and with possible color changes.
   In the weeks following the surgery, it may take 3–4 weeks to have an adequate
   recovery and 3–4 months to obtain the definitive aesthetic and/or functional
   results.

P. Gonzalez-Isaza, R. Sánchez-Borrego (eds.), *Topographic Labiaplasty*,
https://doi.org/10.1007/978-3-031-15048-7

3. Sometimes it is necessary to perform a **second surgical time or revision** to reduce the size of the lips according to the aesthetic conformity and functionality. Most of the time this revision does not generate any type of charge with respect to medical fees, but it could generate minimal operating costs of materials, anesthesia, among others.

4. I agree to limit my physical and sexual activity for as long as indicated by the surgical conditions.

5. I understand that Dr. Pablo Gonzalez Isaza will use all his expertise and knowledge to balance aesthetics, functionality, and conditions but at no time can he guarantee perfect and surreal results.

6. Smoking patients have a higher risk of poor postoperative results and alterations in healing and additionally a greater potential for infectious events and bleeding. **If you are a smoker, it is advisable to stop smoking 2–4 weeks before the surgical procedure,** but this is not a guarantee to avoid the potential complications previously exposed.

7. I certify that I have informed Dr. Pablo Gonzalez Isaza in a timely manner about my medical history and medical background. I understand that withholding information could lead to complications and risks during the surgical procedure.

8. In my own words, the following is what I want to get out of my surgical procedure by Dr: _____
_____
_____
_____

9. I certify, that I have had a consultation with Dr. ------------------------------------ ------------------, and all aspects of my surgical procedure have been properly explained to me.

10. I understand the procedure, its risks, complications, and the recovery process. I agree to carefully follow all the instructions given by Dr. -------------------------- ------------------------ and his team, as well as I will report any eventuality that may occur during the recovery process.

11. I understand that I have received sufficient information in order to make the decision to undergo the surgical procedure. All questions have been answered.

12. Additionally, I authorize Dr. --------------------------------------- to make photographic and video recordings for medical record keeping purposes and may obtain a copy of this material upon request.

13. I authorize Dr. --------------------------------------- a to use photographic and video material related to my surgical procedure, for purely academic and scientific research purposes, preserving at all times my identity and privacy.

_____   _____
Patient Signature   Date

_____   _____
Tutor or assistant   Date

_____   _____
Dr. ------------------------------------- Date

What Do Our Students Think About the Concept of Topographic Labiaplasty?

- **Student 1:**
  It is a comprehensive approach to address all elements to achieve a harmonious and functional result.
- **Student 2:**
  It is a way of speaking the same language; it is a perfect diagramming of the findings, a great idea to achieve perfection in aesthetics.
- **Student 3:**
  It is an excellent way to see the vulva in an integral way; the labia minora and majora are not the only ones, to see it as a whole, with the anatomical variants and cap; it is the best way to achieve an aesthetic and functional result.
- **Student 4:**
  Topographic labiaplasty provides a functional and practical approach to aesthetic vulvoplasty, which makes it the approach to be taken into consideration from now on.
- **Student 5:**
  The topographical labiaplasty classifies the defects by levels and is the best guide that the cosmetic gynecological surgeon has to order the thought and design the surgery attending each part of the external genitalia.
- **Student 6:**
  This concept defines the actual anatomy of a procedure to be performed, a technique that in the prognosis helps to evaluate how to perform a better adequate intervention, for each patient pre- and postsurgical, and its variables.
- **Student 7:**
  The topographical labiaplasty is a concept that gives a global vision and proposes anatomical limits of the female external genitalia, in order to perform a surgical procedure, guided and to obtain a reproducible aesthetic result.

Compedium of Topographic Labiaplasty Images

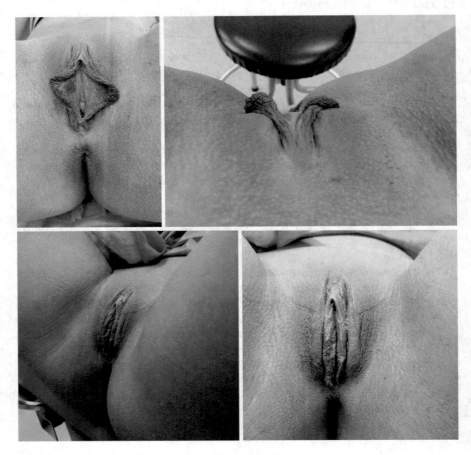

Topographic labiaplasty with anatomical variant approach

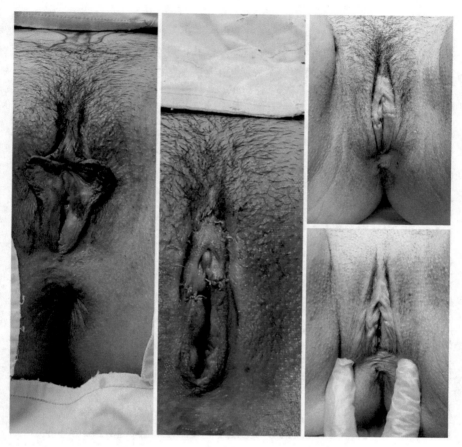

Topographic labiaplasty with asymmetric and aberrant insertion approach of clitoral hood frenulum

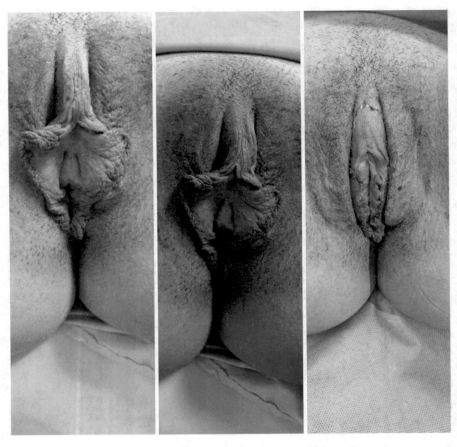

Topographic labiaplasty with multiple anatomical variant approach

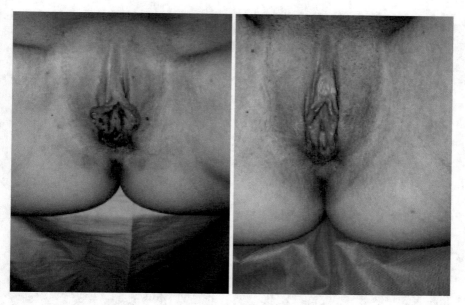

Topographic labiaplasty with anatomical variant approach to the clitoral hood

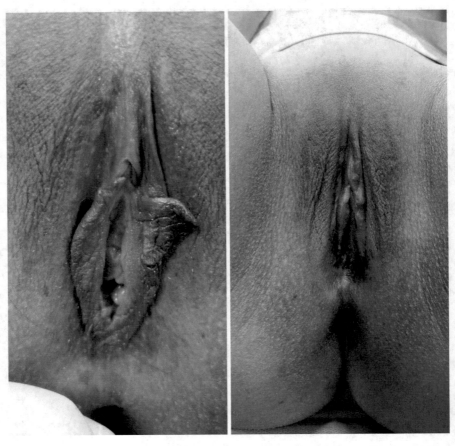

Labiaplasty topographic asymmetry and left anatomical variant approach in the horizontal plane (duplication)

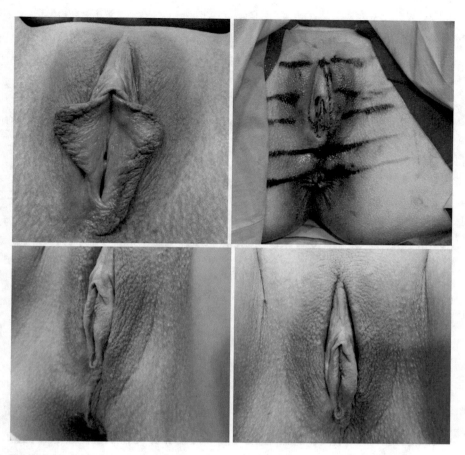

Topographic labiaplasty, anatomical repairs respected, optimal functional, and sexual aesthetic result

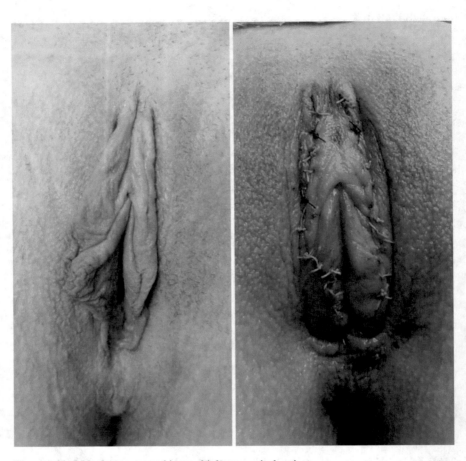

Topographic labiaplasty, approaching multiple anatomical variants

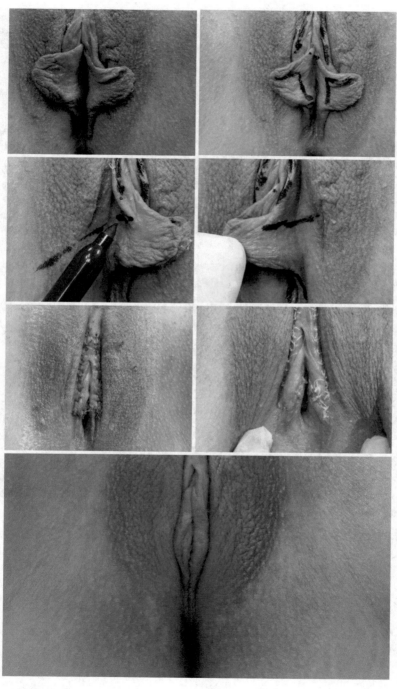

Topographic labiaplasty, approaching multiple anatomical variants, note the importance of an adequate marking of the topographic anatomical landmarks

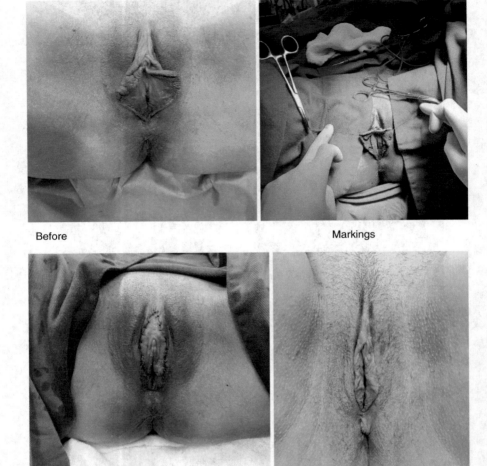

Before   Markings

Inmediate Post Op   Pop 4 years

Labiaplasty, custom flask technique, performed by Dr. Pablo Gonzalez Isaza

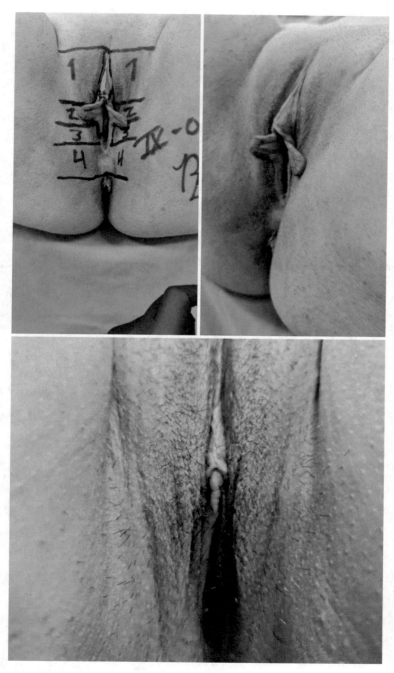

Topographic labiaplasty + clitoropexy, result after 3 months

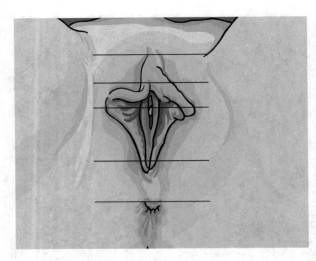

Topographic labiaplasty concept and drawings

Index

Printed in the United States
by Baker & Taylor Publisher Services